HOW TO MARKET HOME HEALTH CARE SERVICES

HOW TO MARKET HOME HEALTH CARE SERVICES

SUSAN D. WILLIAMS, Ph.D., R.N.

Faculty
School of Nursing
University of Missouri—St. Louis
Senior Partner
Williams & Williams
St. Louis, Missouri

JAMES R. WILLIAMS, M.B.A.

Faculty
Management Division
Maryville College—St. Louis
Senior Partner
Williams & Williams
St. Louis, Missouri

WILEY

A Wiley Medical Publication
JOHN WILEY & SONS
New York / Chichester / Brisbane / Toronto / Singapore

Library of Congress Cataloging-in-Publication Data

Williams, Susan D.
　How to market home care services.

　(A Wiley medical publication)
　Includes bibliographies.
　1. Home care services—Marketing.　2. Home care
services—United States.　I. Williams, James R., M.B.A.
II. Title.　III. Series.　[DNLM: 1. Home Care
Services—economics—United States.　2. Marketing of
Health Services—methods.　WY 115 W728h]

RA645.W55　1988　　362.1'4'0688　　87-34098
ISBN 0-471-85887-0

Printed in the United States of America

10 9 8 7 6 5 4 3 2 1

To our parents,
for their support
and editing contributions

Preface

The home health care industry is growing. That should not be news to any home health care practitioner. From 1978 to 1986 the number of hospital-based home health care agencies more than doubled to over 1,000. During the same period, the number of independent home health care agencies grew over 80%. This growth is the result of the tremendous change occurring within the health care industry. Pressures from insurers, employers, and government to reduce health care costs, advances in medical technology, and an increase in patients' sophisticated knowledge about alternative health care have all been a part of this change and a cause of the growth of home health care.

Anyone who has seen a child grow rapidly knows that with growth comes new problems and opportunities. For the child, the problem may only be pants that seem to shrink overnight. For the home health care agency, the growth of the industry has created something new—competition. Henry Ford once said in reference to his Model T, "You can have any color you want, so long as it's black." Nobody complained because the Model T was the only automobile affordable to the middle class. Then the Chevrolet Motor Company introduced a slightly higher priced car in black—and red. Henry Ford didn't sell as many Model T's that year. The lesson Chevrolet taught Ford was that producing a quality product was not enough. Consumers' needs must be identified and satisfied.

Marketing provides a client-oriented focus that forces an organization to identify and meet clients' needs. Home health care agencies must learn how to market effectively if they want to meet their clients' needs—and continue to grow. Using the marketing mix, market plans, and market audits, a home health care agency can define its identity and effectively design the agency's services to better meet clients' needs. Marketing is a tool, when properly used, that will guide a home health care agency successfully into the future.

The purpose of this book is to teach home health care professionals what marketing is and how home health care agencies can use marketing to better meet clients' needs. The book provides step-by-step guidelines to create and implement a successful market plan. Successful marketing examples are taken from the home health care industry. In addition, the book provides an outline of professional sales techniques and successful sales management and motivation. Uniquely, the book also discusses how the administrator can create not only an effective marketing effort, but also an ethical one.

The book is divided into four parts. In Part 1, Chapter 1 discusses what marketing is (and what it is not), how marketing came to be a part of modern business, and what are the pro's and con's to marketing home health care. Additionally, the four "P's" of the marketing mix are discussed. Chapter 2 introduces the reader to some of the traditional marketing concepts: mission, exchange, clients, image/attitudes, target markets, purchase, satisfaction and dissatisfaction, and word-of-mouth advertising. The chapter discusses why each of the concepts is important and how each is used in creating a successful marketing effort.

Part 2 discusses the process by which a market plan is created and implemented. Chapter 3 describes what the market plan is, why a home health care agency needs one, and how a market plan report is created and presented. Chapter 4 discusses the commitment phase of market planning. Included are guidelines for the allocation of budgets and resources and advice for obtaining the commitment of management and staff personnel to the market plan process. Chapter 5 shows how a market audit is conducted. Tools and worksheets necessary for the market audit are included along with instructions for their use. Chapter 6 shows how the completed market audit can be used to identify problem (opportunity) areas. With problem areas identified, goals, objectives, and strategies are created to deal with the problem areas. Chapter 7 explores how strategies are implemented. Chapter 8 shows how the market plan is evaluated and controlled to become a continuous, flexible process by which clients' needs and the agency's competitive environment are constantly being evaluated.

Part 3 shows how the agency's marketing efforts are implemented through marketing communications, professional personal selling, and the effective management of time, sales territories, and sales personnel. Chapter 9 focuses on promotion, particularly communication. Media, channels of distribution, and message development are discussed, showing the home health-care marketer how successful messages are developed. Chapter 10 dispels misconceptions about personal selling and shows how any home health care professional can sell professionally and successfully. Practical keys to successful personal selling are given as is an anatomy of a sales call. The chapter also discusses who should sell for the home health care agency and how those salespeople should be motivated. Chapter 11 illustrates how successful marketers manage their time, their geographic territories, and their salespeople.

Part 4 shows how marketing should fit into the agency's organization and how marketing can be done ethically. The chapters also provide a glimpse of the future and potential markets for home health care agencies. Chapter 12 discusses fitting the marketing function into an agency's organization, selecting a marketing consultant, determining the qualifications of the marketer, and creating an in-house marketing function. Chapter 13 explains classical philosophies of ethics and how the administrator or manager can create a culture of ethical marketing. Chapter 14 looks at the future of home health care and how environmental, political, economic, technological, and demographic factors will effect home health care. Additionally, new opportunities for home health care agencies are outlined.

The authors have strived to provide the reader a practical guide, written in layman's language, to the "mysteries" of marketing home health care. The result of reading and applying the concepts and tools in this book should be a successful marketing effort. And the results of a successful marketing effort should be economic growth for the agency, improved employment security for the agency's employees, and an improved quality of life for the agency's clients.

SUSAN D. WILLIAMS
JAMES R. WILLIAMS

Acknowledgments

We wish to gratefully acknowledge the help and support of colleagues, professionals, and friends who have contributed either directly or indirectly to the creation of this book. Particularly, we would like to single out Janet Foltin, Associate Editor, John Wiley & Sons Publishers, for her patience and perseverance in working with the authors; our colleagues, Dr. Jamie Spikes of the University of Missouri—St. Louis, and Dr. Pam Horwitz of Maryville College—St. Louis for their encouragement and critical thinking on the subject; and Ron Barnes, Executive Director, Missouri Association of Home Health Agencies, for his help in providing ideas and examples for this project. In addition, the authors wish to thank Connie Lacher of the University of Missouri—St. Louis and particularly Portia Simpson of PS and Associates, Clayton, Missouri, for their efforts in typing and revising the manuscript. Finally, we wish to thank friends whose parents needed home health care but who did not know about home care, and thus started us on the idea of teaching home health-care agencies how to better market their services.

Contents

PART 1 MARKETING IN HOME HEALTH CARE:
        WHAT IS IT?   1

1 **WHAT IS MARKETING?**   3

   Brief History of Marketing, 4
   What Marketing Is Not, 5
   Definitions of Marketing, 6
   Marketing Mix, 7
   Pros and Cons of Home Health Care Marketing, 12
   Conclusion, 17

2 **MARKETING CONCEPTS**   21

   Mission, 22
   Exchange, 23
   Clients, 25
   Image and Attitudes, 26
   Target Markets, 32
   Purchase, Satisfaction, and Dissatisfaction, 33
   Word-of-Mouth Advertising, 35
   Conclusion, 36

PART 2   IDENTIFYING AND MEETING CLIENTS' NEEDS: THE PROCESS   39

3   MARKET PLANNING   41

Need for a Market Plan, 42
What Is a Market Plan?, 49
Creating and Presenting a Market Plan Report, 49
Conclusion, 53

4   COMMITMENT PHASE   55

Administration Commitment, 56
Self-Study Tool, 56
Staff Commitment, 57
Budget Allocation, 60
Resource Allocation, 61
Conclusion, 61

5   MARKET AUDIT   63

Market and Market Segments, 65
The Organization, 73
The Client, 77
Competitors, 80
Services and Products, 81
Pricing, 82
Promotion and Advertising, 83
Place, 83
Conclusion, 84

6   PLANNING PHASE   87

Planning Models, 88
Problem Identification, 90
Goals and Objectives, 95
Strategy Development, 96
Conclusion, 99

7 IMPLEMENTATION PHASE 101

Strategies for Implementation, 103
Conclusion, 111

8 CONTROL PHASE 113

Purposes and Types of Evaluation, 114
Data Collection Methods, 116
Criteria for Evaluation, 118
Modification, 123
Conclusion, 123

PART 3 MARKETING YOUR AGENCY EFFECTIVELY: TOOLS AND PERSONNEL 125

9 PROMOTION 127

Communication Process, 128
Channels, 130
Message Design, 132
Marketing Messages, 136
Tools, 137
Conclusion, 145

10 PROFESSIONAL PERSONAL SELLING 147

Five Types of Personal Selling, 149
Three Keys of Successful Selling, 152
The Sales Call, 161
Anatomy of a Sales Call, 168
Final Words on Selling, 173
Selection of Salespeople, 173
Motivating the Sales Force, 174
Conclusion, 174

11 MANAGEMENT OF TIME, SALES TERRITORIES, AND SALESPEOPLE 177

Time Management, 178
Territory Management, 180
Sales Force Management, 183
Conclusion, 185

PART 4 EVALUATING THE ROLE OF THE HOME HEALTH CARE MARKETER 187

12 MARKETING RESPONSIBILITY 189

Organizational Chart, 190
Qualifications of the Marketer, 193
Outside Consultant, 195
In-House Marketing, 197
Momentum, 198
Conclusion, 199

13 MARKETING ETHICS 201

Philosophies of Ethics, 203
Creating Ethical Behavior, 205
Conclusion, 207

14 FUTURE TRENDS IN HOME HEALTH CARE 209

Overall Assumptions, 211
Environmental Changes, 211
Political Changes, 211
Economic Changes, 212
Technological Changes, 213
Demographic Changes, 214
A Future Overview, 215
New Home Health Care Market Opportunities, 216
Marketing Home Health Care and the Future, 219
Conclusion, 219

APPENDIX MARKET PLAN 222

INDEX 233

PART 1

Marketing in Home Health Care: What Is It?

1

What Is Marketing?

Marketing continues to be one of the more controversial terms in health care services today. While all health care providers know they should be doing it, no one is sure what it is. The application of industrial and consumer marketing principles to home health care marketing is so recent that no consensus has yet been developed regarding a definition of marketing that is suitable for all health care providers. Nearly as many definitions of marketing exist as do authors on the subject.

To arrive at a simple but useful definition of marketing home health care, a brief overview of the history of marketing will provide an understanding of the process taking place in the home health care industry today. Because the term marketing is new to the whole health care industry, many misconceptions exist as to what marketing is and what it can do for a home health care agency. This chapter will deal with those misconceptions and provide an accurate set of expectations about the benefits that a marketing orientation can provide the home health care agency. The result of the discussion will be a simple and useful definition of marketing for home health care.

This chapter will also define the term marketing mix and discuss its application to home health care. Finally, this chapter will outline some of the controversy surrounding the application of marketing techniques to health care and home health care in particular.

BRIEF HISTORY OF MARKETING

Unlike health care, which has been studied for ages, marketing is an extremely young discipline. Before the industrial revolution, consumers met their needs, such as food and clothing, by producing products themselves—for example, by slaughtering animals for food and spinning wool for clothing. The industrial revolution began around 1700 in Great Britain (Hodgetts, 1979). The move of the population to cities—and the subsequent specialization of labor and the unavailability of resources, including time, for people to fulfill their needs for food and clothing—created markets, places of exchange, where people could exchange money for goods and services. As markets developed, the merchant class, rose to meet the need for exchanging goods. More important, because of the increased efficiency that factory-produced goods offered, the number of choices available increased rapidly. Furthermore, as people congregated in the cities, their purchasing patterns changed from being tradition directed to being market directed (Mandell and Rosenberg, 1977).

The producers of goods concentrated on fully exploiting their new-found power of production by producing more goods more efficiently. The demand for these products was so new and so high that producers did not have to exert any effort selling, let alone marketing, them. However, as the industrial revolution progressed and competition rose, firms discovered that producing goods was not enough: some sort of sales effort was needed to persuade a prospective customer to purchase one's goods in preference to those of a competitor. Thus rose the sales orientation and the era of the proverbial traveling salesman, or "drummer." The development of a sales effort created industry's first step toward marketing. It is not surprising that many organizations still view marketing as nothing more than an aggressive sales effort.

Following World War II, with production facilities created to support the war effort idled by peace, companies began asking, "What can we do with our production facilities?" Obviously, no consumer demand existed from 150-mm Howitzers or Sherman tanks. To get the answer to the question, businesspeople did something they had never done before. They asked the prospective buyer, "What do you want?" The consumer answered, and plants that had produced bombs began producing baby buggies, and tank plants began producing automobiles. By determining the needs of prospective customers *before* producing, companies created a market orientation. Thus, history indicates that marketing is an orientation towards meeting the needs of the client.

The same progression of thinking has been true for health care. Consider the progress of hospitals over the past century. Initially, the fact that a hospital existed was all that was necessary to fill its beds. As more hospitals were created, they began to sell themselves by focusing on improving the quality of care provided. In the 1980s, hospitals began to take a market-oriented approach by identifying consumers' needs and adjusting to meet them. Home health care has the opportunity to benefit from the experience and mistakes of other health care providers in developing a market-oriented approach to their service.

WHAT MARKETING IS NOT

First, marketing is not selling. Selling is a part of marketing, but marketing is more than just selling—just as all cows have four legs, but not all four-legged things are cows. Yet the terms are often used interchangeably and erroneously. The misconception exists that marketing is a more sophisticated or more genteel form of selling.

This difference in the common perception of marketing and selling can be simply illustrated. Imagine that your child, a college senior, has returned home for Christmas break. She or he proudly announces the decision to make a career in sales. What would be your reaction? Probably, you would question your child's judgment or even your ability as a parent. Where did you go wrong? In contrast, what if the announcement had been that your child would seek a career in marketing? More than likely, your thought would be, "Well, it's not nursing, but at least it isn't selling." Ironically, but possibly, part of the confusion between marketing and selling may have started in the early 1970s when companies, to avoid sexist terms, chose to refer to those involved in sales as marketing representatives rather than salesmen or, more awkwardly, salespersons. Regardless of where or how misuse of the term marketing started, to market the services of a home health care agency successfully, one must do more than be able to sell.

Hospitals have provided prime examples of the misinterpretation of marketing and misplaced expectations of the application of marketing principles. Hospitals began to move toward a marketing orientation when they began to realize that just being there or being able to provide high-quality care was not enough to fill all the beds. The solution appeared to be public relations. The thinking was that the better people thought of the facility, the more likely they would be to utilize its services. It was also assumed that the public relations department would be able to keep a positive image, regardless of the facts, in front of the public. Hospitals with this approach to marketing have been sorely disappointed with the results they have received. And the reason is simple: while public relations is a part of marketing, marketing is more than just public relations.

The same is true with hospitals' recent entries into advertising. Hospitals, as well as home health agencies, that rely on advertising as their entire marketing effort will be disappointed with the results. Advertising is a part of marketing, but marketing is more than advertising.

DEFINITIONS OF MARKETING

Several respected authors have provided definitions of marketing that are useful for those who produce services:

Marketing is the analysis, planning, implementation and control of carefully formulated programs designed to bring about voluntary exchanges of values with target markets for the purpose of achieving organizational objectives. It relies heavily on designing the organization's offering in terms of the target markets' needs and desires, and on using effective pricing, communication, and distribution to inform, motivate and service the markets.

—Kotler, 1975: 6

Marketing is a bridge linking the organization with its external environment, orienting it toward customers and other constituencies, and helping management to position its efforts in relation to competitors. Marketing is analysis, planning, organizing and control of carefully formulated programs set in the context of long-term goals and objectives.

—Cavusgil, 1986: 72

Health care marketing management is the *process* of understanding the needs and wants of a target market. Its purpose is to provide a viewpoint from which to *integrate* the organization, analysis, planning, implementation, and control of the health delivery system.

—Cooper, 1985: 3

For marketers of home health care, we believe the following definition of marketing suffices. Marketing is the process or mind set that focuses the agency's efforts and actions on identifying and meeting the clients' needs and wants. While the primary purpose is to meet clients' needs, a secondary goal is to enhance the exchange of client and agency values.

Hence, the primary purpose of marketing is to serve clients. To identify and meet the needs and wants of clients and to prepare the home health care agency to meet those needs, a marketing mix must be developed.

MARKETING MIX

Kotler (1984: 68) provides the following definition of the marketing mix: "marketing mix is the mixture of controllable market variables that the firm" (agency) "uses to pursue the sought level of sales in the target market." McCarthy (1981) first identified and categorized those uncontrollable market variables and labeled them the four Ps: product, price, promotion, and place (or distribution). Since McCarthy originally developed the four Ps for an industrial product setting, some modifications are necessary to discuss marketing services such as home health care. The combination of those variables is unique for every organization, just as a set of fingerprints is unique to an individual. It is the marketing mix that differentiates your agency from any other organization offering competitive services.

Every organization must differentiate itself from competitors. After all, if your service is no different than another's, why would a consumer choose your agency instead of the other? The marketing mix is the tool to create the differentiation. Home health care agencies do not offer to the public a tangible product such as an automobile. Rather, an agency's product is the combination of services offered. In part, the marketing mix of your agency is determined by the services you offer. Does your agency offer a complete line of home health care services, such as homemaker services, high-tech infusion therapy, food service, and physical or occupational therapies? By defining or even deciding what services your agency offers, you have begun to differentiate your agency from others.

Price has a unique place in the marketing of health care services. Purchasing health care services is unlike the purchase of a new automobile, where a prospective consumer may purchase one care over another because of a price difference of less than 1%. Patients or clients rarely haggle over price of health care before the purchase. Have you ever heard a client say, "I want to feel $250 better" or "just do a double bypass; I can't afford the quadruple you recommend." No other product or service is more expensive and less price sensitive.

The role of price in the marketing mix is based in microeconomic theory. Microeconomics concerns the relationship between demand and supply and between costs and profit. In a perfectly competitive market—a theoretical condition that does not exist in reality—the supply of a service equals the demand for the service at a market price. However, the demand (how much of a service is wanted) is related to the price of the service. For example, if a dentist charged $100 for cleaning your teeth, how often would you have your teeth cleaned? However, if the dentist charged $10 for the same service, would you use the service more or less frequently than if the price was $100? The term price elasticity, or price sensitivity, describes the relationship between price and quantity sold, or demanded. The relationship is expressed as follows:

$$E = -\frac{\%\ \Delta Q}{\%\ \Delta P} = -\frac{\Delta Q/Q}{\Delta P/P} = -\frac{\Delta Q}{\Delta P} \cdot \frac{P}{Q}$$

where

E = coefficient of price elasticity
Q = quantity demanded
P = price
Δ = change in

Figure 1.1. *Price elasticity is defined as the relationship between price and quantity sold.*

If the value of E is greater than 1, demand is elastic. A given percentage change in price will result in a greater percentage change in quantity demanded. In other words, a small price change results in a more significant change in quantity demanded (Ferguson, 1978).

However, if the value of E is less than 1, demand is considered inelastic. If demand is elastic, total revenues from a service will rise if the price is lowered. If demand is inelastic, total revenues will decrease if the price is lowered. It should also be noted that elasticity can be measured only for relatively small changes in price. A service that exhibits elasticity at one price level may exhibit inelasticity at another.

Another unique attribute of health services pricing is the presence of third-party payers. What kind of a car would you buy if your bank expected only a portion of the money borrowed to be repaid? Third-party payers in many situations remove the consumer, that is, the client, from directly dealing with price. Home health care is unique in the health care field in that it has the opportunity to utilize price in its marketing mix. Some agencies have built their business exclusively on Medicare reimbursements, while others purposefully avoid government involvement in reimbursement. Home health care does utilize all three methods of reimbursement, third party, direct pay, and Medicare-Medicaid. Therefore, it would seem unlikely that a home health care agency would be successful if the following advertising campaign was launched: "Christmas special: five visits in one week only $200! Offer valid only with coupon and through December 25." However, to those paying the agency, price can be a point of differentiation between your agency and the competitor.

Promotion is the P that most people think of when they think of marketing. Promotion includes all the activities of promoting one's agency, including advertising, personal selling, public relations, and sales incentives. Promotion is perhaps the least attractive of marketing Ps to health care practitioners. Some feel that any health care that must be sold must be of questionable quality. However, promotion is extremely important to the success of any business. The rhetorical question has been asked, If a tree falls in the forest and no one is around to hear it, does it make a sound? Similarly, for clients to use your services, they first must know that the services are available. Two ways exist for an agency to provide information about their services to prospective or future clients. One way is marketer dominated; the other way is termed, simply, other (Engel et al., 1986). The difference is whether you as the marketer can control the message being transmitted to prospective clients, your target market. Perhaps the clearest example of a marketer-dominated channel is advertising. In advertising, the marketer is paying for the opportunity to have a specifically designed message reach a specific target audience.

In contrast, other typically refers to word-of-mouth advertising. No advertising or promotion is more effective than word-of-mouth advertising. Word-of-mouth advertising occurs when one person tells another about a product or service or recounts their experience or that of a friend with a particular firm. When was the last time you told a friend, "I like shopping at Sears, because . . .," or conversely, "You wouldn't believe how long I waited for service at Joe's Market." Word-of-mouth advertising takes the form of personal recommendations, and therein lies its effectiveness. Any consumer is more likely to use or try a product or service when a trusted friend has recommended it (Richins, 1984). Also, word-of-mouth advertising is remembered much better than other forms of advertising. While you personally may have the attitude, "I don't care what people say about me," such an attitude regarding your business or livelihood can be extremely dangerous. Studies (Engle et al., 1986) have shown that a satisfied customer will tell about eight people about a positive experience. However, 80 people will hear of the experience of a dissatisfied customer! The lesson for the importance of client relationships should be clear. Marketer-dominated areas of promotion are discussed in detail in Chapter 9.

In consumer goods and industrial markets, the fourth P, place (or distribution) refers to where the product is made available to the target market and how the product gets to the target market from the place of manufacture. For home health care agencies, place has two meanings in the definition of the agency's marketing mix. First, place refers to the geographic location of the agency. The location of the agency is a factor in determining the target market of the agency. For example, prospective clients in Minneapolis will probably not be a target market for an agency whose only location is St. Louis. Likewise, an agency located in Newark, New Jersey, a part of metropolitan New York, may be unable to provide services in western Connecticut, also a part of metropolitan New York.

The second meaning of place for home health agencies is where the service is delivered to the client. Obviously, this is the client's home. One of the unique features of home health care is that it is the only form of professional health care available to the patient in his or her own home.

Developing a marketing mix for an agency is critical to the success of the agency. Describing an agency's marketing mix is no different from describing yourself or a friend. Just as in a description of yourself, the focus should be on what makes you unique, the same is true for an agency's marketing mix. However, many service organizations, such as home health care agencies, have had difficulty in thinking in terms of the four Ps: product, price, promotion, and place. After all, the four Ps, which were developed in the 1960s, used traditional industries as the model. With the recent growth of the service sector of the economy, more thought has been given to applying traditional marketing concepts to the needs of a service-based firm.

Magrath (1986) has recently proposed that seven Ps be used in the development of a marketing mix for service firms. In addition to the traditional product, price, promotion, and place, Magrath has added personnel, physical facilities, and process management. Magrath (1986: 48) states: "*Personnel* are key to the creation of the service and its delivery to the consumer in a consistently acceptable fashion. [Clients] identify and associate the trait of . . . personnel with the traits of the firm" with whom the service personnel are employed. This is particularly true with home health care agencies, where the service is provided in the home, away from the agency's physical assets. It is possible that the client's only contact with the agency is the person rendering aid. Therefore, for the home health care agency, not only is the selection of qualified personnel important; the professional appearance and demeanor of employees in contact with clients are also critical to the image and marketing efforts of the firm. Indeed, if the home health care agency is to maximize its probability of success, the professionalism of employees should actively be developed and managed.

Regarding physical assets, Magrath (1986: 48) states: "A consumer must experience a service. This experience is greatly affected by both the setting that is visible to the customers and the physical assets hidden from view." Magrath uses as an example Disneyland's physical appearance coupled with its infrastructure (machinery, maintenance, etc.), which is invisible to visitors. For a home health care agency, just because services are delivered exclusively in the client's home does not mean that the physical office facility can be run-down, neglected, or disorganized. For example, Domino's Pizza, whose business is exclusively home delivery of pizza, maintains neat facilities decorated in bright colors. Why? It is human nature to assume that if the facility producing the product or service is shabby, the shabbiness is automatically reflected in the quality of the service. This does not mean that a home health care agency must have offices with prestigious addresses. It does mean that wherever the offices are located, the facilities must be neat and well maintained in order to provide quality services and to avoid creating a negative image of the services offered.

According to Magrath (1986: 49), the "seventh P, process management, involves the task schedules, routines, and supervision of activities" conducted in preparing and delivering the services. Industrial firms have operations management that concentrates on improving the efficiency of producing goods; the home health care agency can differentiate itself from competitors by the efficiency with which it handles clients' needs and the ability with which it predicts those needs in advance.

Regardless of the number of Ps, the marketing mix is what sets one home health care agency apart from another. The components of the marketing mix are what makes a prospective client select your agency in favor of another. Failure to pay attention to the marketing mix has the same result as going through life without ever looking in a mirror. The image an agency has of itself may be entirely different from how others see it. The market audit (Chapter 5) outlines the details of how the marketing mix is identified and modified to meet the needs of clients.

PROS AND CONS OF HOME HEALTH CARE MARKETING

Before 1970, the words marketing and health care could never be found used together. Indeed, the study of marketing in any context did not begin until after World War II. Therefore, it is not surprising that controversy still rages, particularly in the health care arena, as to the value and even the ethics of marketing.

Pros

The reality of today's health care world is that possessing the ability to provide quality health care is not sufficient to guarantee an adequate livelihood for one's family or those of employees. Today's world is one of limited resources. Marketing helps improve the odds that your agency will be able to earn its fair share of those dollars. Levinson (1984: 26) succinctly promotes "ten truths of marketing you must never forget":

1. The market is constantly changing.
2. People forget fast.
3. Your competition isn't quitting.
4. Marketing strengthens your identity.
5. Marketing is essential to survival and growth.
6. Marketing enables you to hold on to your old customers.
7. Marketing maintains morale.
8. Marketing gives you an advantage over competitors who have ceased marketing.
9. Marketing allows your business to continue operating.
10. You have invested money that you stand to lose.

These truths constitute the pros of—or reasons for—marketing. Each of these reasons will now be discussed in terms of the home health care administrator.

The Changing Market

Simply look at the differences in home health care today compared to that of just 10 years ago. As long as our economy remains capitalistic, innovation and change—looking for a better way—will be with us throughout the future. Marketing is the ear to the ground that, for those who listen, provides the assurance that the organization will be able to meet the challenges of the future. Without marketing, some people might still be sitting around wondering why their fine, high-quality buggy whips are not selling.

People Forget

The consumer is wise and sovereign; that is, the customer is always right. In addition, the increasing amount of information available to the consumer is making the consumer more sophisticated about the alternatives available, particularly in the area of health care. However, that same increase in information is constantly cluttering the consumers' minds and making recall of any message, including yours, more difficult. To allow a client to select your agency, your agency's name must be in the consumer's mind when the consumer recognizes a need for your service. Marketing helps keep your agency's name in the consumer's mind. More specifically, marketing keeps your solution to the consumer's problem available so that the consumer can take the action you desire.

Your Competition

There are people in this world who want your job. There are people who want the food on your table. Almost everybody, if given the choice of feeding themselves or feeding someone else, will choose feeding themselves every time. Simply put, if you do not take care of your agency and your clients with proper marketing, someone else—namely, your competition—surely will.

Agency Identity

Your agency's identity is embodied in your reputation and reliability. Marketing forces one to guard that reputation constantly and to make the changes necessary to maintain or improve that image. Differentiation (the four Ps) is what makes your agency different from others. The differentiation is the basis for your agency's identity.

Survival and Growth

The history of American business is littered with examples of product and business failures that were the result of a lack of marketing or improper marketing. Polaroid Corporation's Polavision (instant slides) and Ford Motor Company's Edsel are two notable examples. Both were technological advances, but they were created without input from the intended market. Home health care agencies that focus solely on quality of care or any one aspect of the business run the risk of sharing the same fate of the Edsel.

Does proper marketing assure survival and growth? No. However, the lack of proper marketing virtually ensures that the agency's life or business will be curtailed or develop less than its full potential.

Keeping Established Customers

For home health care agencies, keeping established customers does not mean that an agency should continue to provide services to clients after the need for the services has passed. What it does mean is that any agency's best source of new clients is previously satisfied clients. For the home health care agency, previous clients include both the people who received the services and those who may have been involved in arranging the service, such as discharge planners or referring physicians. A part of human nature is to choose that which is familiar and that which previously satisfied a need. Marketing can help keep your agency's name and services positively in the minds of previous users. The result is that when such people need services similar to yours, they will think of you first. Also, if a friend or an acquaintance of a satisfied, properly marketed client needs your service, your satisfied client will effectively promote your agency for you.

Morale

Marketing, when properly done, should make one feel good. Why? Because through marketing you are essentially listening to your clients' needs. Everyone should have the experience of holding a conversation with an excellent listener. It feels good. Listening to a client's needs is treating that person with respect; moreover, it places value on their opinions. In addition, promotional tools such as advertisements can be motivational reminders to the agency's employees of the image and reputation they are charged with maintaining. When you look in the mirror, don't you stand a little straighter? The same effect occurs when members of an organization see the messages that are communicating the organization's image and goals to outsiders.

Competitors Who Do Not Market

Levinson (1984) points out that you should continue to market regardless of economic conditions. Businesses typically reduce marketing expenditures, including advertising, when business declines. Such action only increases the tendency for revenue to decline in recessionary times. What bigger advantage can an agency have other than listening to their clients? Agencies that do not market are not listening to their clients.

Continuing Business

Marketing does not guarantee commercial success, just as accurate accounting or good clinical skills do not guarantee the success of a home health care agency. Marketing helps your agency by communicating the benefits your agency offers clients and prospective clients. Also, marketing keeps your agency attuned to the changing needs of clients. Both of these actions substantially enhance the probability that your agency will be able to continue operating.

Protecting Your Investment

Regardless of whether you are an employee of an agency or a principal of the agency, you have money and time at stake. For the employee, regular income is jeopardized by being employed by a failing firm. Moreover, being associated with an unsuccessful concern is not considered martyrdom when seeking a new employer. For the owner, the risks may be even greater than for the employee. After all, the money and time you have invested in the agency is at risk. It is exactly this increased risk for the owner that should dictate a commitment to a marketing orientation and plan.

Cons

The reluctance of health care professionals to discuss marketing probably stems from both a misunderstanding of what marketing is and the American Medical Association's (AMA's) long-standing prohibition against members' advertising. In 1847, the AMA stated in its code of ethics, "It is derogatory to the dignity of the profession to resort to public advertisements . . . inviting the attention of individuals afflicted with particular diseases" (American Medical Association, 1847). Court rulings over the years have caused the AMA to modify its prohibition, and today the AMA's code of ethics reflects the ethics of the Federal Trade Commission and the advertising industry in general. The AMA's official opposition to marketing is now limited to focusing on the "creation of unrealistic expectations" (MacStravic, 1986: 286). Marketers of home health care may find that remnants of this attitude may still exist, particularly among the uninformed and misinformed. Agencies that actively market may have to suffer the disdain of those who consider such activities as unprofessional. However, those health care providers who do not market have a slim chance of existing in the future.

Marketing costs money. Often the positive results of successful marketing cannot be directly tied to expenditures. Indeed, the elimination or absence of marketing expenses can create improved short-term financial results. Therefore, it is possible for an agency that does not market to have superior financial performance compared to one that is actively investing in the future through marketing expenditures. However, such results are short-lived and illusory. Too often, particularly in recessionary times, marketing expenditures are viewed as discretionary. Although marketing costs money, it need not be expensive and should be viewed as a critical investment with benefits far outweighing the costs.

Marketing costs time. Marketing takes personnel away from the core purpose of the agency: providing health care services in the home. (In a law or accounting firm, the statement would be that marketing reduces billable hours.) Any organization must conduct activities other than its main purpose of producing and delivering services. Statements must be prepared, bills sent, bills paid, deposits made, and lunches eaten. Each of these activities could be said to take time away from the core purpose of providing services. However, each of these activities is required if the organization is to continue to exist. The same is true for home health care marketing. The investment of time in marketing is an investment in the future of the agency.

Marketing is not a panacea or prescription for commercial success. Overly optimistic expectations of the results of improper marketing can create crises, disappointments, and even financial ruin when such predictions are not fulfilled. Marketing should be an integral part of operating a successful commercial organization. Marketing is no more or less crucial to the success of a venture than is accurate bookkeeping or technical competence.

Specific outcomes of marketing cannot be predicted reliably. Marketing is not a hard science like chemistry. In chemistry, the result of the reaction between two compounds is certain and predictable, conforming to the immutable laws of nature. The only certain result of sound marketing actions is that the likelihood of a successful outcome is improved.

CONCLUSION

Marketing is a relatively new concept, appearing in the industrial sector only after World War II. The application of marketing theory is newer yet, particularly when applied to the increasingly service-oriented economy. Home health care agencies are uniquely positioned to take advantage of and apply the concepts of marketing.

Marketing must be an integral part of any successful commercial enterprise. Marketing provides a client-oriented focus that forces the organization to identify and meet clients' needs. Through the use of the marketing mix, organizations can define their identity and effectively design their offering to better meet clients' needs.

Debates and objections continue over the place marketing should have in health care organizations. Misconceptions and inaccurate information still exist as to what marketing is and what it can do for an organization. The principles of marketing, when properly applied and executed, create a positive, responsive attitude that puts the client's needs, rather than the provider's convenience, first.

Good marketing cannot guarantee commercial success, but it does substantially enhance the probability of success. Virtually every commercial failure in the history of American business can be traced to a lack of good marketing—the lack of identifying and meeting the prospective clients' needs.

REFERENCES

American Medical Association Code of Ethics. New York: H. Ludwig & Co., 1847. New York: H. Ludwig & Co.

Cavusgil, S. T. Marketing's promise for hospitals. *Business Horizons.* 29 (September–October 1986):71–76.

Cooper, P. D. *Health Care Marketing: Issues and Trends* (2nd ed.). Rockville, MD: Aspen, 1985.

Engel, J. F., Blackwell, R. D., Miniard, P. W. *Consumer Behavior* (5th ed.). Chicago: Dryden Press, 1986.

Ferguson, C. E., Maurice, S. C. *Economic Analysis: Theory and Application.* Homewood, IL: Irwin, 1978.

Hodgetts, R. M. *Management: Theory, Process and Practice* (2nd ed.). Philadelphia: W. B. Saunders, 1979.

Kotler, P. *Marketing Management* (5th ed.). Englewood Cliffs, NJ: Prentice-Hall, 1984.

Kotler, P. *Marketing for Nonprofit Organizations* (2nd ed.). Englewood Cliffs, NJ: Prentice-Hall, 1975.

Levinson, J. C. *Guerrilla Marketing.* Boston: Houghton Mifflin, 1984.

MacStravic, R. E. S. *Managing Health Care Marketing Communications.* Rockville, MD: Aspen, 1986.

Magrath, A. J. When marketing services, 4 P's are not enough. *Business Horizons.* 24(May–June 1986):44–50.

Mandell, M. I., Rosenberg, L. J. *Marketing* (2nd ed.). Englewood Cliffs, NJ: Prentice-Hall, 1977.

McCarthy, E. J. *Basic Marketing: A Managerial Approach* (7th ed.). Homewood, IL: Irwin, 1981.

Richins, M. L. Word-of-mouth communication as negative information in *Advances in Consumer Research*, vol. 11. Kinnear, T. C. (ed.). Provo, UT: Association for Consumer Research, 1984, 697–702.

2

Marketing Concepts

Before an effective market plan can be created for a home health agency, several concepts of the core theory of marketing must be discussed. The marketing mix was discussed in Chapter 1. The need for and role of mission, exchange, clients, image, purchase, satisfaction, dissatisfaction, and word-of-mouth advertising are discussed in this chapter.

MISSION

Would you take a cruise on a boat that did not have a compass? Would you go on a cross-country automobile trip without a road map? Of course not. Yet, attempting to operate a home health care agency or any enterprise without a mission statement is just as dangerous as sailing without a compass or driving without a road map.

A mission statement provides a "long-term vision of what the agency is striving to become. Ideally, mission statements are couched in terms narrow enough to provide practical guidance, yet broad enough to stimulate creative thinking" (Crompton and Lamb, 1986: 53). A well thought-out, written mission statement provides everyone in the organization, particularly those working independently or remotely, such as home health care personnel, with a "shared sense of purpose, direction, significance, and achievement" (Kotler, 1984: 49). The mission statement communicates the organization's reason for being to managers and employees. With the mission of the agency clearly stated, managers can more easily formulate goals and objectives that are congruent with the agency's mission and purpose. Indeed, before a home health care agency can develop an effective market plan, the mission of the agency must be defined.

Creating a mission statement can be as simple as answering the question, "What business are we in?" Management consultant Peter Drucker states, "Few companies have any clear idea of what their mission is and that is one of the . . . major causes of their worst mistakes" (Hampton, 1986: 140). Flexner, Berkowitz, and Brown (1981: 13) suggest that the mission statement comes from "balancing the answers to four fundamental questions":

1. What (services) do we want to provide? (What businesses do we want to be in?)
2. What will we be allowed to do?

3. What do we have the resources to do?

4. What does society need?

Some examples of mission statements in the health care field are the following:

> The mission of the American Red Cross is to improve the quality of human life; to enhance self-reliance and concern for others; and to help people avoid, prepare for and cope with emergencies. It does this through services that are governed and directed by volunteers and are consistent with its congressional charter and the principles of the International Red Cross.
>
> —American Red Cross 1985 Annual Report

> Humana, Inc., provides an integrated system of health care services that includes hospital care, prepaid health care and indemnity insurance plans, and medical care centers where independent physicians deliver primary medical care. In responding to the needs and values of patients, physicians, employers, and working people, Humana provides high-quality health care at affordable prices.
>
> —Humana, Inc., 1986 Annual Report

> At Baxter Travenol, we seek to offer the best products, systems and services to health-care providers around the world, enabling them to deliver quality care more efficiently. To realize this goal, we will:
>
> —provide quality and value in the goods and services we offer our customers;
>
> —establish and maintain leadership positions in the health-care markets we serve, and
>
> —promote an environment for employees that fosters teamwork, personal growth and respect for the individual.
>
> Achieving these objectives will serve health-care needs worldwide and increase the value of our stockholders' investments.
>
> —Baxter Travenol, Inc., 1985 Annual Report

EXCHANGE

According to Kotler (1984: 8) exchange is the "act of obtaining a desired product" (or service) "from someone by offering something in return." Exchange is one of four ways by which a person may satisfy needs and wants. The other three ways are self-production (the satisfaction of a need or want with no interaction with anyone else); coercion (the satisfaction of a need or want by force); and begging (the satisfaction of a need or want by requesting the voluntary, unrewarded release of resources). Note that only in the process of exchange is something of value traded for something different of equal perceived value.

Five conditions must be present for exchange to take place (Kotler, 1984: 8):

1. There are at least two parties.
2. Each party has something that might be of value to the other party.
3. Each party is capable of communication and delivery.
4. Each party is free to accept or reject the offer.
5. Each party believes it appropriate or desirable to deal with the other party.

Bagozzi (1975) has identified three types of exchange: restricted, generalized, and complex. Each has implications for marketers of home health care.

Restricted exchange involves only two parties and is symbolically represented by A $\leftrightarrow$ B where $\leftrightarrow$ means gives to and receives from. Restricted exchange is characterized by a great deal of effort to maintain equality, a quid pro quo mentality, and short time intervals involving the mutual reciprocities (Ekeh, 1974). Restricted exchanges are the simplest variety, such as one finds in making a retail purchase. For home health care agencies, restricted exchanges occur when recipients of home health care services arrange and pay for the services themselves.

Generalized exchange involves at least three participants and is represented by A $\rightarrow$ B $\rightarrow$ C $\rightarrow$ A. Here, $\rightarrow$ represents gives to. In generalized exchange, the participants benefit, not directly, but indirectly. In retailing, a consumer buying a product or service with a credit card is as an example of generalized exchange. The credit card issuer actually pays the retailer; the customer pays the credit card issuer, and the customer receives the desired good. In home health care, generalized exchange typically involves third-party payers: the client receives services which are paid for by another party.

Complex exchange may be either straight or circular in shape. Complex exchange refers to a system of mutual relationships among at least three parties. Using the same model, complex circular exchanges are represented by A ↔ B ↔ C ↔ A, while complex chain exchanges are represented by A ↔ B ↔ C. In reality, most exchanges are complex because of the involvement of more than two parties and the numerous benefits that are exchanged. Even in the simplest example involving a client paying money in exchange for home health services, more than just money and services enter into the exchange.

What is involved in exchanges with home health care agencies and the agency's clients? Obviously, the home health care agency provides services such as nursing and homemaking services, and the client provides money in exchange for those services. That description, however, does not adequately describe the total exchange relationship. The client may also be receiving comfort in being in his or her own home, peace of mind because of not being in a hospital or nursing home, and the companionship of other family members and pets. Ireland (1986) suggests that home health care agencies offer patients care, comfort, coping, credibility, and curing. The exchange relationship between agency and client involves more than just money and services. Identifying and knowing the elements involved in the exchange can help agencies understand the benefits they provide clients.

Does the client offer more than money to the agency as part of the exchange relationship? While certainly, in most cases, the agency expects to receive money for services rendered, the client may also provide excellent recommendations; additional business through referrals to friends or acquaintances (also known as word-of-mouth advertising); or, if conditions warrant, repeat business through requesting your agency. A client can even provide an agency's personnel the satisfaction of a job well done or reinforcement of professional images.

CLIENTS

Clients are an integral part of the marketing process for any business organization. Obviously, no business can exist long without clients. Clients start the exchange process by using services provided by the home health care agency. More important, clients determine the services desired and the value of those services. The adage "the customer is always right" has been translated into consumer theory, which states that the consumer is sovereign. As mentioned in Chapter 1, spectacular failures have occurred when "experts" have attempted to force ideas, products, or services on unwilling consumers by underestimating or ignoring the client's sovereignty.

Where does client sovereignty come into play with a typical home care situation in which the arrangements for care have often been made on behalf of a patient by a hospital's discharge planner or directed by a medical doctor? Unless a patient is under the legal guardianship of another, under legal age, or is non compos mentis, every patient has the legal right to refuse medical care. A home care patient can refuse care or request that another home care agency provide service. In either case, the client has exercised sovereignty. The result is that the home health care agency that ignored the client's sovereignty has lost a client, revenue, and the opportunity to improve the client's life by providing care.

The role of the client cannot be overemphasized. The successful marketing efforts of a home health care agency—which will have a significant impact on the success of the agency—*must* center on identifying and meeting the clients' needs and wants. The client not only provides the agency with revenue that will ensure an ongoing business but also provides the critical information needed to adjust the agency's offering to meet customer needs better and to survive and grow over the long term.

IMAGE AND ATTITUDES

Someone has said that reality does not count; perception of reality is what is really important. This does not mean that the role of image in home health care marketing is a matter of deceit and trickery. Rather, positive image communicates that your agency provides reliable, quality care.

Have you ever heard an audio tape recording of your own voice? Did you recognize it? Did it sound the way you thought it should? Most people can recognize their own voice, but very few people sound the way they expected. Why? We have an image, a perception, of our voice. Until we hear a recording, the perception we have is reality. However, the tape recording is undeniably an accurate reflection of reality. Is there a difference? Which voice do others hear coming from our mouths: the one on the tape or the one in our perception?

Can you describe the qualities of your home health care agency? Does your perception of your agency match that of people outside your agency? Successful image management in home health care marketing assures that the perceptions of clients match your own. Clients are more likely to purchase services that have a positive image (Assael, 1984). A successful image can create opportunities and reduce the possibility of losing opportunities.

Successful image management requires three steps: measuring the image, monitoring or maintaining the image, and modifying the image.

People's attitudes toward a product, service, or company result, in part, from their beliefs about the product, service, or company. Attitude is made up three components: cognitive (one's beliefs), affective (one's likes or dislikes), and conative or behavioral (one's actions or behavior) (Engel et al., 1986). Attitude can more simply be defined as what clients "know, feel, and do" (Seattle and Alreck, 1986: 119). To illustrate the differences among the three components, consider the following example. A consumer could honestly make all of these statements about a hypothetical home health care agency: (1) "XYZ Home Health Care Agency has the most professional staff" (cognitive); (2) "I don't like XYZ Home Health Care Agency because they employ male nurses" (affective); (3) "I haven't used XYZ Home Health Care Agency because I haven't been ill in the past 10 years" (behavioral). Note that these statements are not mutually exclusive. More important, each statement could be made in response to a questionnaire and yet each would give a different picture of the client's view of the agency.

Attitudes (and an agency's or service's image) are learned and enduring and have direction and potential (Settle and Alreck, 1986). Direction and potential are particularly important in the United States as our culture has a definite tendency toward twofold moralizing, that is, we view everything as either good or bad with no categories in between. Because attitudes are learned, marketers have the opportunity to influence that learning process, which will be discussed later.

Attitudes are influenced by family, peer groups, information, experience, and personality (Assael, 1984). Social class, cultural values, religious values, and ethnic considerations can also influence attitudes (Engel et al., 1986). The effective marketer must consider all of these influences when designing a service to meet clients' needs or attempting to measure the image of an agency.

Measuring one's image can be as simple or complicated as one's need for complete and accurate information. For example, a simple but effective method is used by Mayor Ed Koch of New York City. When Mayor Koch walks down the street, he constantly asks people, "How am I doing?" By informally tallying positive versus negative responses, the Mayor has a reasonable idea of peoples' attitudes toward him as well as a gauge of his current image. Most significant, he is able to discover changes in attitudes quickly.

More complicated, in-depth methods exist using multiattribute attitude models analyzed with multivariate statistical techniques. Well over 40 separate models exist for measuring attitude (Wilkie and Pessemier, 1973). Typically, such analyses are conducted by full-service market research firms and can be useful in developing a detailed diagnosis of an agency's strengths and weaknesses. Most models are based on or are modifications of Fishbein's model (Fishbein, 1967; Ajzen and Fishbein, 1980). At the risk of oversimplifying, Fishbein's model states that attitude toward a behavior (such as using home health care services) is the sum of beliefs that a particular behavior will result in a particular consequence, modified by the relative importance of that particular consequence.

To see how the model can be used, see Figure 2.1. Data are developed using a Likert-type scale where a selected population is asked to comment on various beliefs about, for example, home health care. For instance, to develop a perception of the attitudes about home health care, the questions in Figure 2.1 might be asked.

Note that in Figure 2.1 the scales reverse occasionally to prevent respondents from routinely marking one column. (Marketing research practice is to discard as invalid responses that are the same for every question.) The scales can be designed to meet your own needs. To determine the clients' attitudes, simply sum the values of the responses according to topic, such as price perception or attitude toward your agency.

The information you can generate about your agency and its image is limitless. You must decide what you want to find out. An initial image measurement tool can be developed by yourself, with others, or by a professional market researcher. Most important, any survey tool must be pretested (critiqued by a small number of those who will be the target of the survey) to ensure that the messages you intend are the messages being communicated.

One important point to consider in measuring beliefs and attitudes is the role inferential beliefs play in consumers' attitudes toward

If I were ill, I would prefer to be at home rather than in a hospital.
Definitely not _____ : _____ : _____ : _____ : _____ : _____ : _____ Definitely
$\qquad$ −3 $\quad$ −2 $\quad$ −1 $\quad$ 0 $\quad$ +1 $\quad$ +2 $\quad$ +3

Nurses employed by (your agency) are competent.
Strongly agree _____ : _____ : _____ : _____ : _____ : _____ : _____ Strongly disagree
$\qquad$ +3 $\quad$ +2 $\quad$ +1 $\quad$ 0 $\quad$ −1 $\quad$ −2 $\quad$ −3

Having a hot meal prepared in my home by a home health care service costs more than $25.
Definitely _____ : _____ : _____ : _____ : _____ : _____ : _____ Definitely not
$\qquad$ −3 $\quad$ −2 $\quad$ −1 $\quad$ 0 $\quad$ +1 $\quad$ +2 $\quad$ +3

Only rich people can afford nursing care in their home.
Definitely _____ : _____ : _____ : _____ : _____ : _____ : _____ Definitely not
$\qquad$ −3 $\quad$ −2 $\quad$ −1 $\quad$ 0 $\quad$ +1 $\quad$ +2 $\quad$ +3

I can afford nursing care in my home.
Definitely _____ : _____ : _____ : _____ : _____ : _____ : _____ Definitely not
$\qquad$ +3 $\quad$ +2 $\quad$ +1 $\quad$ 0 $\quad$ −1 $\quad$ −2 $\quad$ −3

Figure 2.1. Model for measuring attitude.

products and services. In other words, absence of information never prevents a consumer from giving an opinion. Consumers will use whatever information is available—even none—to form an opinion. Most important, to that consumer, opinion is fact until overwhelmingly proven otherwise.

To understand the prevalence of inferential beliefs, consider how you would respond to the following statement:

Ronald Reagan will go down in history as the most effective United States president of the twentieth century.
Strongly agree _____ : _____ : _____ : _____ : _____ : _____ : _____ Strongly disagree
$\qquad$ +3 $\quad$ +2 $\quad$ +1 $\quad$ 0 $\quad$ −1 $\quad$ −2 $\quad$ −3

Most people, including yourself, would have no trouble in providing an answer to that question. Yet, in actuality, only scholars of United States presidential history would be qualified to give an accurate answer. Your responding to this example demonstrates the existence of inferential beliefs. Inferential beliefs have a significant impact on actions, such as your vote in an election, using the example.

Once the initial image measurement has been made, the image must be monitored for any unfavorable changes. The agency's image can be monitored intermittently or constantly. Preferably, the agency should do both.

Intermittent image measurement involves measuring the agency's image on a routine basis, be it quarterly, semiannually, or annually. Typically, the same survey tool used to initially measure the agency's image can be used. Slight modifications or improvements in the tool can be made to focus on issues raised in the earlier survey. The results of the more recent survey should be compared with earlier surveys to determine in what areas the image has changed significantly and in which direction (better or worse) the image is moving.

Intermittent measurement has the advantage of allowing for a more exhaustive, in-depth measurement of image, particularly if the results are analyzed for response by given target markets. However, intermittent measurement has the significant disadvantage of the length of time passing between measurements. If surveys are conducted on an annual basis, the risk is that a significant—and unrecognized—deterioration of the agency's image could have occurred during that year.

As stated earlier, the client is sovereign. However, consumers can also be fickle. Consumers' attitudes can change rapidly and dramatically. Therefore, home health care agencies should constantly monitor their image, regardless of whether intermittent measure is planned.

Constant measurement of the agency's image can be simple and economical. One method is to conduct an interview with the patient, the patient's family members, the referring physician, and/or the discharge planner following the closure of the case. The interview can be conducted in person, by telephone, or through a mail survey. Results can be plotted, and trends over time can be noted.

Constant monitoring also can aid in identifying dissatisfied clients. When a dissatisfied client is identified, the source of dissatisfaction should be investigated and, if necessary, remedies proposed. Remedies can take the form of dealing with the client's dissatisfaction by refunding monies, offering an apology, or simply listening and paying attention to the client's complaint. Remedies can also take the form of changing policies, procedures, communications, or even personnel to correct the situation that caused the dissatisfaction.

The importance of constantly monitoring clients' views and attitudes, which make up the image of the agency, cannot be overemphasized. First, a majority of dissatisfied customers never complain to the organization with which they are dissatisifed (Shuptrine and Wenglorz,

1981). Most important, a sincere effort on the part of the organization to discover the problem, discuss the problem, and attempt to rectify the problem results in a clear improvement in satisfaction (Harmon and Resnik, 1982). The power of word-of-mouth advertising was discussed in Chapter 1. To maintain an agency's positive image and word-of-mouth advertising, a constant monitoring of the agency's image is absolutely necessary.

What happens if the image of the agency as reported by surveys is different from the image the agency desires? If the image is less desirable than the agency wants, clearly a need exists to modify the image. However, the first step in modifying an image must be to recheck one's data, survey tools, and analyses to find out if any of these could have caused the unexpected results. Also, the environment in which the image measurement was conducted also needs to be examined for unrelated but influential factors. For example, while the survey measuring all agency's image is being conducted, local news media may focus attention on a crime allegedly committed by an employee of another home care agency. Such a problem can be compounded when agencies have similar names or have failed to differentiate themselves in the eyes of the public.

The second step is to determine why the agency's image is less than desired. Is it a matter of misinformation about the agency, as in the preceding example? Is it because of bad experiences with a particular employee or a particular policy? Such questions can be answered through another survey that focuses on the area of concern.

Another method of finding out why an agency's image is less than desired is to conduct focus groups of potential or past clients. Focus groups are guided group discussions usually lead by a trained group leader. The group leader leads the conversation to cover subjects of interest to your agency. Focus groups allow a more in-depth discussion of issues than do surveys. Ideally, the focus group leader is not an employee of your agency and the focus group session is conducted away from your agency's premises. Focus groups can provide insight as to how your agency earned its image.

Some adverse images are relatively simple to change. For example, an image of low quality might be successfully changed by requiring those in contact with the public to adhere to a dress code of nurse uniforms or other appropriate business attire. An image of unfriendliness might be changed by providing training in telephone etiquette to those who answer the phones.

However, a critical point must be made about changing or modifying the image of one's agency. Superficial changes designed to enhance the agency's image must be backed by concrete facts. A professional dress code may enhance the image of the quality of care an agency provides, but the cleanest, most crisply pressed uniforms will not change the agency's image if care is being given by incompetent people. The most sophisticated marketing techniques cannot make a silk purse out of a sow's ear.

Measuring, monitoring, and modifying the agency's image provides the opportunity to ask target markets, "How am I doing?" Most important, the process provides the agency the opportunity to learn from the experience. Recognizing the need to measure, monitor, and manage clients' attitudes toward one's agency and the image of the agency necessitates a discussion of target markets.

TARGET MARKETS

If your agency has a single location in Pittsburgh, should you be concerned about the attitudes of consumers of home health care agencies in Tacoma, Washington? Probably not. Right now in the United States alone there are over 250 million potential users of your agency's services. (This is a conservative estimate of the country's population.) Do you want to have all of them as clients? Can you provide service to all 250 million? Probably not. Therefore, a need exists to limit the population (i.e., create a target market) to a number or description your agency can reasonably serve.

In developing a market plan (see Chapter 3), creating your target market plays an important role in defining the needs of your potential clients. Target markets can be defined just about any way you choose. Establishing geographical limitations is usually reasonable. Likewise, your agency can target paying methods (private pay versus third-party payers), age of client (pediatrics versus geriatrics), or level of care (high-tech versus custodial).

The use of target markets focuses your agency's attention on the needs of those most likely to use your services and away from those who are least likely to use them. An agency can have multiple target markets. By defining target market needs, your agency can differentiate among the needs of potential clients and tailor its communication to that target audience. For example, if you define a target market as the elderly in a given geographic area, your communication might emphasize quality of care or the improved quality of life of being in one's own home as opposed to a hospital or nursing home; or the communication might promote a spouse's day out by providing services to allow a spouse who cares for an infirm partner the benefit of an afternoon out shopping. In contrast, if your target audience consists of couples with young children, you would want to communicate how your services could provide sick-day care, allowing a working parent to avoid missing work.

Defining target audiences allows you to communicate more effectively. For example, you do not talk to a 5-year-old the same way you talk to an adult because they have different levels of comprehension and attention. Put another way, you do not bite into the rind of a watermelon and continue munching until the watermelon is gone. You slice the watermelon into manageable pieces so that you can attack the desirable parts while avoiding the less attractive ones, such as the rind. Such are the advantages of selecting target markets.

PURCHASE, SATISFACTION, AND DISSATISFACTION

When a decision maker decides to use your agency's services and communicates that decision to your agency, a purchase has been made. (Some may say that a sale is not complete until the money is collected. However, for this discussion, only the marketing implications of purchase are being considered.) Managing purchase and its outcomes is part of the ongoing marketing process since clients are a major source of both positive and negative information about your agency and the services you provide.

Who the decision maker is will be discussed more fully in Chapter 10; but in terms of making the purchase, the decision maker can be the person who will receive your services, a discharge planner, or a referring doctor. When that person makes the decision and communicates the decision to the provider, the decision maker has weighed the costs and benefits of using your services versus those of using other home health care agencies and versus using none at all. The benefits that purchasers perceive come from their own beliefs, attitudes, and intentions as well as from you, the marketer.

Individual characteristics, social influences, and situational influences play a part in the decision process. Individual characteristics include the decision maker's (1) personality, (2) motives, (3) values, and (4) life-style. Social influences include (1) normative influences, or "conforming with the expectations of others to attain or avoid outcomes controlled by others" (Engel et al., 1986: 306); (2) cultural and ethnic influences; (3) reference or peer group pressures; (4) family influences; and (5) religious influences. Situational influences include (1) physical surroundings; (2) social surroundings; (3) task definition, or goals; (4) temporal perspective, or time pressures; and (5) antecedent conditions, such as moods or the assignment of a patient to a home health care agency (Belk, 1974).

Purchase has two outcomes: satisfaction and dissatisfaction. Satisfaction is the evaluation that the chosen alternative confirms prior beliefs and expectations. Dissatisfaction occurs when that confirmation does not take place (Engel et al., 1986).

A client is satisfied when beliefs about your agency's services are confirmed and when expectations about the benefits are met or exceeded. More important, the decision to use your agency is positively reinforced (Assael, 1984). Positive reinforcement increases the likelihood that the action of using your agency will be repeated. If the satisfied decision maker is a referring physician or discharge planner, the agency can expect to be given increased referrals or priority in assigning clients.

A concern that has been expressed in many forums is that marketing any form of health care might create demand for unneeded or even unhealthy medical procedures. (e.g., "I think I'll have an appendectomy this month because it's on sale. Nothing is wrong with my appendix now, but it'll probably have to come out sooner or later.") The supposed risk is that if a home health care agency successfully satisfies the needs of a client, that client may continue to request services after the medical justification for the service has passed. In actuality, unneeded services or products are rarely sold by ethical marketers. Indeed, virtually every industry has examples of clients whose requests for products and services were turned down because, in the opinion of the supplier, the product or service would not meet the needs of the client. Such an action can have the benefit of creating a loyal client. The goal of ethical, successful marketing is not to create the unneeded use of a service, but rather to generate loyalty so that when the service is needed, your agency's name is thought of first.

A satisfied client will tell other people, some of whom may be prospective clients, about the positive experience. Discharge planners may share their success with others at professional meetings. During a Wednesday afternoon of golf, referring physicians may tell peers about their positive experiences or their patients' positive experiences with your agency. This is word-of-mouth advertising, the most powerful type of advertising available. Word-of-mouth advertising is so powerful because it takes the form of personal recommendations. If you are hiring a home health care nurse and have a choice between two equally qualified persons, you would probably be more likely to hire the one recommended by a trusted friend. In such cases, the person hired has benefited from positive word-of-mouth advertising. However, word-of-mouth advertising can be negative when clients' needs and expectations are not met.

The other outcome of a purchase is dissatisfaction—when clients' expectations are not met. Dissatisfaction results in a reduced likelihood of repeat purchases. In addition, dissatisfaction creates negative word-of-mouth advertising. Moreover, dissatisfied clients are more likely to tell others about their negative experience than satisfied clients are to discuss their positive ones. For example, think of the last time you personally had a positive experience at a retailer. How often have you told the story of your positive experience to others? Now think of a negative experience involving a retailer. Which experience did you tell to others more often? Dissatisfied former clients may be telling others about their negative experience about your agency right now.

Most dissatisfied clients do not tell the person or agency that caused the dissatisfaction about their dissatisfaction. So how can an astute marketer monitor word-of-mouth advertising? The most useful, most important method is to routinely survey clients' and decision makers' attitudes following the completion of the service. If dissatisfaction is discovered, it can be dealt with in two ways. First, if the dissatisfaction is a result of misunderstanding, discussion may clarify the issue and remove the misunderstanding, thereby improving the likelihood of a repeat purchase. Second, if the dissatisfaction is the result of procedures or personnel, internal actions, such as revising procedures or replacing or retraining personnel, may be necessary to prevent the recurrence of dissatisfaction.

WORD-OF-MOUTH ADVERTISING

If word of mouth is so powerful and not directly controlled by marketers, can it be managed? The answer is yes. Word-of-mouth advertising can be influenced through good public relations by keeping a positive image before the public in newspapers, on television, and in local magazines and by creating positive personal experiences through community activities, such as volunteering personnel for blood drives, health fairs, or televised fund-raising auctions.

Another way of creating positive word-of-mouth advertising is to identify and influence (i.e., inform) opinion leaders about your services. Opinion leaders are "individuals who exert either directly (e.g., face-to-face communications with others) or indirectly (e.g., through others observing their market-related behaviors) a significant amount of social influence" (Engel et al., 1986: 315). What would be the effect on your agency's level of business if the president of the local branch of the American Medical Association in a speech singled out your agency as an example of excellent care and cooperation in carrying out doctors' orders? Even though that person may have had no first-hand experience with your agency, the person was nonetheless functioning in the role of opinion leader. Opinion leaders can be identified and informed—"wooed"—concerning the benefits your agency's services. People in positions of professional leadership are usually opinion leaders. For home health care services, opinion leaders might be respected physicians and hospital administrators, directors of nursing and discharge planners who are active in professional organizations, or leaders of the local chapter of the American Association of Retired Persons (AARP) or senior citizen community centers or groups.

Opinion leaders can also be created. For example, department stores create opinion leaders among teenagers by inviting one from each area high school to participate on a teen fashion advisory board, and the stores sell more clothes in the process. Likewise, a home health care agency could create opinion leaders by designating an advisory board of respected, recognized members of the target market, such as senior citizens, discharge planners, pediatric physicians, and so on.

CONCLUSION

Your agency's mission statement gives direction and purpose to the efforts of you and your people. Identifying target markets focuses your agency on likely users of your home health care services. Understanding the exchange process helps to identify the benefits your clients and your agency receive as a result of providing home care services. Measuring, monitoring, and managing the image of your agency help create a positive predisposition in prospective clients toward your agency. Remembering that the client is always right and knowing the costs—in terms of negative word-of-mouth advertising—of ignoring that adage forces your agency to take a client-focused, market-oriented approach to operating a home health care agency. Taken together, these concepts form a framework around which a thorough marketing audit and a prescription for business success can be built.

REFERENCES

Ajzen, I., Fishbein, M. *Understanding Attitudes and Predicting Social Behavior.* Englewood Cliffs, NJ: Prentice-Hall, 1980.

American Red Cross, Inc. Annual Report, 1985. Washington, DC.

Assael, H. *Consumer Behavior and Marketing Action.* Boston: Kent, 1984.

Bagozzi, R. P. Marketing as exchange. *Journal of Marketing.* 39(October, 1975):32–39.

Baxter Travenol, Inc. Annual Report, 1985. Deerfield, IL.

Belk, R. W. An exploratory assessment of situational effects in buyer behavior. *Journal of Marketing Research.* 11(1974):156–163.

Crompton, J. L., Lamb, C. W. *Marketing Government and Social Services.* New York: John Wiley & Sons, 1986.

Ekeh, P. P. *Social Exchange Theory: The Two Traditions.* Cambridge, MA: Harvard University Press, 1974.

Engel, J. F., Blackwell, R. D., Miniard, P. W. *Consumer Behavior* (5th ed.). Chicago: Dryden Press, 1986.

Fishbein, M. A. A behavior theory approach to the relations between beliefs about an object and the attitude toward the object in *Readings in Attitude Theory and Measurement.* Fishbein, M. (ed.). New York: John Wiley & Sons, 1967.

Flexner, W. A., Berkowitz, E. N., Brown, M. *Strategic Planning in Health Care Management.* Rockville, MD: Aspen Systems Corp., 1981.

Hampton, D. R. *Management* (3rd ed.). New York: McGraw-Hill, 1986.

Harmon, R. R., Resnik, A. J. Consumer complaining: exploring expected and desired responses in *An Assessment of Marketing Thought and Practice.* Walker, B. J. (ed.). Chicago: American Marketing Association, 1982, 175–178.

Humana, Inc. Annual Report, 1985. Louisville, KY.

Ireland, J. Marketing for Home Care. Conference of the Missouri Association of Home Health Agencies. Kansas City, MO: December 9, 1986.

Kotler, P. *Marketing Management* (5th ed.). Englewood Cliffs, NJ: Prentice-Hall, 1984.

Settle, R. B., Alreck, P. L. *Why They Buy: American Consumers Inside and Out.* New York: John Wiley & Sons, 1986.

Shuptrine, F. K., Wenglorz, G. Comprehensive identification of consumers' marketing place problems and what they do about them in *Advances in Consumer Research*, vol. 8. Monroe, K. B. (ed.). Ann Arbor, MI: Association for Consumer Research, 1981, 687–691.

Wilkie, W. L., Pessmier, E. A. Issues in marketing's use of multi-attribute attitude models. *Journal of Marketing Research.* 10(November 1973):428–441.

PART 2

Identifying and Meeting Clients' Needs: The Process

3

Market Planning

One of the keys to good marketing is developing a sound market plan. Market planning encompasses analysis, planning, implementation, and evaluation of marketing programs.

NEED FOR A MARKET PLAN

Planning is essential if home health care agencies are to meet the challenges of the rapidly changing health care market. Saxena (1985) suggests that market planning provides an agency with these additional benefits:

1. Stimulates thinking to use resources
2. Assigns responsibilities
3. Sets schedules
4. Coordinates efforts
5. Facilitates control and evaluation
6. Creates awareness of obstacles
7. Identifies marketing opportunities
8. Provides information sources
9. Leads to achieving agency's goal

Each of these nine benefits will now be examined to determine what it means to the home health care administrator.

Stimulating Thinking

In today's market of limited resources, everyone needs to stimulate their thinking beyond the services they currently offer and to expand their scope. Ask yourself such questions as: What resources do we have in our staff that are not being utilized? What resources are not available in the marketplace? Are there any other services in our community that could be added to our agency for better service to the customer? Is the agency using all available resources—such as consultants, staff, literature, laws, and leaders in the field—to help predict where the agency should be in the future?

Early home health agencies and visiting nurse associations provided one service: nursing care. By stimulating their thinking, home health agencies of today have multiservices, durable medical equipment companies, and profit arms. Ireland (1986) defines this as one-stop shopping, a concept that evolved from examining and using available resources. This type of agency is profiled in Table 3.1.

Assigning Responsibilities

The second benefit of a market plan is that it assigns responsibility. No matter how large or small the agency is, responsibility for coordinating the development of a market plan should be assigned to an individual. It is best if a market plan is not done by one person but based upon the input of many. Different people will add different ideas and expand the market plan to better serve the agency.

Depending on an agency's size and financial resources, it may hire a consultant to develop the plan, assign the marketing director the

---

**Table 3.1   The New Home Health Agency:
One-Stop Shopping**

Skilled care
   Home nursing care
   Diabetes
   Ostomy
   Maternity
   Physical, occupational, and respiratory therapy
   Intravenous therapy
   Speech therapy
Respite and companion care
Homemaker services
Mobile diagnostic services
Pharmacy
Durable goods
Corporate health
   Health screenings
   Health promotion and wellness
   Employee health services
   Employee physicals
Health Education
Case management and social service
Contract services
Videotape rental
Sick child care

---

responsibility, or make it a total staff responsibility. Whatever method is chosen, some mechanism should be established to have staff input into the total plan.

Setting Schedules

The benefit of any plan usually means accountability for time. Assigning the responsibility of the market plan also means that deadlines are set so the plan is accomplished according to the schedule. Having a schedule of how to meet the changing health care system will allow the agency to be prepared for change—not simply to react to it.

Coordinating Efforts

A market plan also provides a means for an agency to coordinate its efforts in the development of its market. Too often, one group within an agency does not know what the other group is planning. The market plan requires an in-depth look at the internal and external environment of an agency to determine how all the services work together to better service the client's needs. Having one person accountable for coordinating the plan also increases the coordination of efforts among departments or different services.

Control and Evaluation

Controlling and evaluating are two of the critical benefits of market planning. Kotler (1982) describes the purpose of marketing control as maximizing the probability that the organization will achieve its short-run and long-run objectives in the marketplace. The purpose of evaluation is to judge whether the organization is performing optimally from a marketing point of view (Kotler 1982). By controlling and evaluating, the agency can respond appropriately and in a timely manner to the many surprises in the implementation of the market plan and modify it as necessary.

Obstacles

Being aware of obstacles facing the agency or program allows the agency to deal with them head on. Many times the administrator or a certain staff member is aware of obstacles but others are not. Putting the obstacles down on paper helps everyone in the agency to become aware of the obstacles and help think of solutions. Examples of obstacles might be regulations, too few personnel, a staff that is unprepared to deliver high-tech services, and increased competition.

Marketing Opportunities

Identifying marketing opportunities is one of the more exciting benefits of a market plan. Staff can brainstorm new ideas about how to better serve the client. In identifying market opportunities, it is important to build on the trends in the marketplace but also to forecast the future. Predictions on the future can be made through a simple process of keeping abreast of trends by reading journals, newspapers, and industry and trade publications, and tracking general trends in the marketplace. For example, diagnosis-related groups (DRGs) have been implemented in the hospital setting, and will probably be applied to home care in the future.

There are also very sophisticated and costly methods of forecasting, such as the Trend Impact Analysis (TIA), which was first developed by the Futures Group, in Glastonbury, Connecticut (Buell, 1986). The approach to developing a TIA forecast is threefold: (1) estimates are made of the probability that a given event will have taken place by one or more specific future dates; (2) estimates are made of the length of time between the occurrence of the event and both its first impact and its maximum impact; and (3) estimates are made of the maximum impact that occurrence of the event would have. A large number of individual forecasts are then generated using random combinations of assumptions.

Predictions of the future can be simple or complex. The important element is that predictions of the future be done consistently in order to be prepared for the new trends.

Information Sources

Market planning involves identifying, utilizing, and bringing together information to facilitate planning. Information can be obtained from formal and informal sources. Some examples of formal sources are books, annual reports, government reports, and trade journals. Informal sources include your staff, professional associates, friends, and clients. Specific sources for information are listed below.

Formal Sources

Books
  Sorkin's Directory of Business and Government
  Directory of Associations
  Statistical Abstracts of the United States
  Health United States
  Advertising Age Yearbook
  Prevention 86/87
  Life Insurance Fact Book
  National Health Directory

Annual reports from
  Hospitals
  Holding companies
  Insurance companies

Corporate reports
  Issues in Home Care, Laventhol & Horwath
  Health Care at Home, Shield Healthcare Centers
  Handbook about Care in the Home, AARP

Chamber of commerce reports

Telephone directories
  National directory of 800 numbers
  National directory of addresses and telephone numbers
  City business directories

Government reports from
  National Center for Health Services Research
  Health Care Financing Administration
  United States Department of Health and Human Services
  Office of Disease Prevention and Health Promotion

Directory of health and social services published in major cities

Journals
  Caring
  Home Health Journal
  Home Healthcare Nurse
  Nursing Economics
  Hospitals
  National Association of Home Care Report
  Home Care
  Home Care Consumer

Home Health Care Services Quarterly
Journal of Health Care Marketing
American Journal of Public Health
Nursing Outlook
Nursing and Health Care
Health Marketing Quarterly

Newsletters
Hospital Product Line Report
Communication Briefings
Hospital Guest Relations Report
Home Care Marketer
Health at Home
Home Health Line
Home Care Clinical Director's Newsletter
Healthcare Marketing Report
Hospital Home Health
Services Marketing Newsletter
Health Care Marketer

Informal Sources

Your staff

Professional associations
National Association of Home Care
National Center for Home Care Education and Research
National League for Nursing
American Hospital Association
American Nurses' Association
American Public Health Association

Hospital councils

Foundations
Foundation for Hospice and Home Care

Health planning groups, state and national level

Your friends

Receptionists of potential or existing clients

Your clients

Service clubs

Community colleges and universities

Agency Goals

The last benefit of a market plan is that it leads the agency to achieve it's goals. Robinette (1970) comments that planning cannot proceed until the end result, or goal, has been decided upon. The selection of the goal is always a subjective, judgmental process. Planning, therefore, is a thoughtful process, and thinking is an important kind of action.

Typically, the health planning model used in health organizations has been to state specific goals, develop strategies to achieve the goals, implement the strategies, and then evaluate the whole process. Marketing literature provides a different planning model. The consumer—a physician, patient, discharge planner, or other purchaser—is recognized as the focal point for making the key choices that will direct the organization's success. In this model (Berkowitz and Flexner, 1978) the consumer is considered in the beginning of the planning process. Consumers then can be grouped into different market segments, such as elderly, new mothers, or pediatrics. Figure 3.1 illustrates the difference between the two planning approaches.

In the market planning model, the initial planning includes an in-

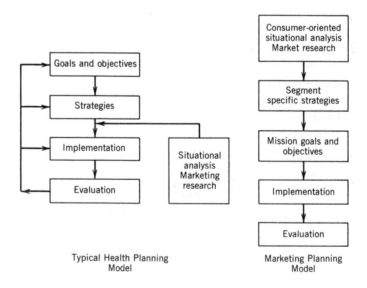

Figure 3.1. *Two planning models. (Source: Berkowitz, E., Flexner, W. The marketing audit: a tool for health service organizations.* Health Care Management Review 3(4) 1978:52–53. *Reprinted with permission of Aspen Publishers, Inc.,* © *1978.)*

depth analysis of the organization by means of a market audit to determine what internal capabilities the organization has to meet the need of its clients or potential clients. Strategies are then developed for each particular segment of the market. Then specific goals and objectives and the strategies for achieving them are defined. These strategies are carried out and the program is implemented. Evaluation is then done to see if the program reached the desired goal and to determine what modifications might be needed.

Traditionally, health organizations have planned services without regard to the consumers' needs and wants. A market planning approach lets the consumers' needs and wants guide the strategy of the organization.

WHAT IS A MARKET PLAN?

A market plan is a continuous process concerned with five phases:

1. Obtaining commitment from management to carry out a market plan
2. Carrying out an audit of the internal and external environment
3. Formulating plans to identify problem areas and develop strategies to achieve goals
4. Implementing and monitoring the strategy
5. Instituting control to evaluate performance and modify the plan

Carrying out each phase develops the total market plan for the agency. Figure 3.2 demonstrates the continuous process of the market plan and the feedback loop.

The appendix shows the complete tool for carrying out a market plan. Each step of this plan will be discussed in detail in Chapters 4–8.

CREATING AND PRESENTING A MARKET PLAN REPORT

A plan doesn't just happen. A system to create a market plan must be designed to meet the agency's requirements. How the system is designed will depend on the amount of skill and information available. Remember, the marketing plan is a continuous process that can be added to quarterly, yearly, or at whatever interval the agency sets up. As experience is gained, the market plan will reflect this through more detailed information and strategies.

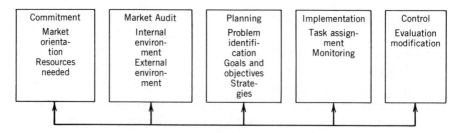

Figure 3.2. *The market plan process.*

Someone has to be responsible for developing the initial plan. This can be done by a marketing director, a marketing committee, a consultant, or all of the staff. Kotler and Bloom (1984) remind us of the maxim that planning should be done by those who must carry out the plans.

The final marketing plan report has seven components: executive summary, background information, objectives and goals, marketing strategies, the scope of work, budget, and controls (Kotler, 1982). Each of these components will now be discussed individually.

Executive Summary

The executive summary is a brief overview of the market plan. It explains why the marketing audit was conducted and lists the major conclusions and recommendations (Morris and Fitz-Gibbon, 1978). The executive summary is designed to give a quick overview of the marketing efforts and should be no more than one to two pages long.

Background Information

Next, the market plan report gives background information obtained from the marketing audit. This material summarizes prevailing conditions and other important observations. For example, data on the activity of the agency would be appropriate:

1. Income from
   Medicare
   Medicaid
   Private pay

Third party

2. Number of visits

3. Number of denials

4. Major types of clients

5. Major services rendered

Nursing

Physical therapy

Occuaptional therapy

Speech therapy

Nutrition counseling

6. Source of referrals

Following these data, which show the pattern of agency usage, a description of trends or major developments in the profession should be given.

Opportunities and threats facing the organization should be described next, and they should be realistic. Opportunities and threats are usually factors that affect the organization from the outside, such as new competitors, new regulations, a shortage of nurses, or cash flow problems.

Strengths and weaknesses should then be listed. The list of strengths helps identify the base on which to build strategies, while the list of weaknesses allows the agency to recognize items that need correcting. For example,

Strengths

1. Twenty-four-hour service, comprehensive services

2. Adequate staff for general services

3. Income from three different sources

Weaknesses

1. Additional staff needed for highly skilled nursing care

2. Public unaware of our services

Objectives and Goals

Setting objectives and goals involves looking ahead and describing the desired future of an organization (Crompton and Lamb, 1986).

Specific goals and objectives should be set that reflect the desired future in operational terms. This list should contain, not wishes, but very specific attainable goals.

Marketing Strategies

Next, the market plan report describes the actual strategies that will be implemented. Information is included about the rational for each strategy and the steps or procedures necessary to carry it out.

Scope of Work

A chart should detail the tasks that need to be undertaken, including the resources needed, sequence, and due dates of each task. Due dates can be specified by week, month, or year, depending on the complexity of the model. This type of graphic display is referred to as a Gantt chart (see Figure 3.3).

Budget

Based on the goals, objectives, and strategies the agency has selected, the budget is presented. The budget should include a detailed account

Task	Resource	Month						
		1	2	3	4	5	6
1. Present marketing plan to management	Report and John Brown, director of marketing	→					
2. Task 1			→				
3. Task 2			→				
4. Task 3				→			
5. Task 4					→		
6. Final report						→	
7. Monthly summary of activities				→			

Figure 3.3. Gantt chart for planning.

of direct labor costs, other direct costs, labor overhead rate, general and administrative expenses, travel expenses, profits or fees, and total project cost (Connor and Davidson, 1985).

Controls

The last section of the market plan report describes the system of controls that have been developed. A control system is established to maximize the probability that the short- and long-term objectives of the agency will be met.

The goals and objectives of the program will direct the way controls are established. The control phase concerns whether and how well the objectives and goals were achieved. After these questions are answered, the agency will know what actions must be taken to improve the results.

CONCLUSION

One of the keys to good marketing is developing a sound market plan. Some of the benefits planning provides an agency are that it stimulates thinking to use resources, assigns responsibilities, coordinates efforts, identifies opportunities, and leads an agency to achieving its goal.

Traditional health planning models were developed to state specific goals and to work toward those goals. In contrast, marketing literature provides a planning model that is developed around the consumer's needs and how the agency can meet those needs. In the latter market planning approach, the consumer's needs and wants guide the strategy of the organizaiton.

The market plan consists of five phases: commitment of management audit, problem identification, strategy development, strategy implementation, and evaluation and modification of the plan.

Once this process has been completed, it is summarized in a market plan report that includes seven parts: executive summary, background information, objectives and goals, marketing strategies, the scope of work, budget, and controls.

The process of developing the market plan clearly helps the agency develop its best strategies for meeting the needs of its clients.

REFERENCES

Berkowitz, W., Flexner, W. Marketing audit: a tool for health services organizations. *Health Care Management Review.* 13(1978):51-57.

Buell, V. *Handbook of Modern Marketing* (2nd ed.). New York: McGraw-Hill, 1986, 46-52.

Connor, R., Davidson, J. *Marketing Your Consulting and Professional Services.* New York: John Wiley & Sons, 1985.

Crompton, J., Lamb, C. *Marketing Government and Social Services.* New York: John Wiley & Sons, 1986.

Ireland, J. Marketing for Home Care. Conference of the Missouri Association of Home Health Agencies. Kansas City, MO: December 9, 1986.

Kotler, P. *Marketing for Non-Profit Organizations.* Englewood Cliffs, NJ: Prentice-Hall, 1982.

Kotler, P., Bloom, P. *Marketing Professional Services.* Englewood Cliffs, NJ: Prentice-Hall, 1984.

Morris, L., Fitz-Gibbon, D. *How to Present an Evaluation Report.* Beverly Hills: Sage Publications, 1978.

Robinette, T. What is health planning? *American Journal of Nursing.* 18(1970):33-35.

Saxena, S. Why, What and How of Market Planning. Seminar on Marketing Strategies and Planning for Medical Professional Services, American Marketing Association, St. Louis Chapter. St. Louis: October 21, 1985.

4

Commitment Phase

For a market plan to be successful, the commitment phase is one of the most important steps. If there is not commitment initially from the administration, the market plan will not be accepted or highly utilized.

Ireland (1977: 58) has commented that an agency "should begin with a genuine commitment from the administration to invest a specific amount of money and staff resources. Marketing should be viewed as an investment rather than an expense that will help optimize the capacity and ability of the agency to effectively respond to the needs of its market segments."

ADMINISTRATION COMMITMENT

Commitment must come not only from the administrator of the agency but also from the board of directors, advisory boards, or investors, depending on the type of home health care agency. Harry Gardner, chairperson of the board of trustees of Northwestern Hospital in Chicago, (Walter, 1981: 92) commented that "particularly now, with the increasing complexity of our institutions, I feel that it is important for the Board to periodically step back and look at the hospital from a variety of perspectives. A marketing study is an attempt to achieve this type of understanding. The results of this kind of measurement can be invaluable in helping define strengths as well as weaknesses and in providing direction for future programs."

It is important to determine whether the administration is committed to both developing and implementing a market plan. There is nothing more frustrating than to produce a report and then have it sit on the shelf. This commitment should be assessed early in planning.

SELF-STUDY TOOL

Van Doren and Smith (1985) have developed a tool to use with boards of directors and other members of the administration to gain an understanding of the need for and relevance of market planning. This tool (Table 4.1) can be used by an administrator or marketing person to help facilitate better communication and understanding of marketing in the organization. By going through the questions in Table 4.1, members of the administration will be able to determine the extent of their organization's marketing orientation.

The tool was developed to be used by nonprofit agencies. Marketing efforts by nonprofit agencies involve contributors to their agency as well as its clients. Contributors can be charitable organizations such as United Way, corporations, associations, and individuals. This marketing tool can be adapted for use by profit-making agencies by simply deleting questions about contributions.

The self-study is divided into four sections, and a five-point rating scale is used. A low score on the orientation section indicates that the organization is unclear about the markets it is trying to reach and the benefits it offers to the public.

Low scores on the research questions indicate that planning is often based on assumptions, not on documented facts obtained through research. Low scores in market planning show that very little long-term planning is done; rather, the organization takes a project-by-project approach.

Low scores in marketing control indicate that there is little evaluation or feedback regarding the services an organization offers.

A score of 80-100 indicates that the organization has very good marketing abilities, a score of 60-79 good abilities, and a score of 40-59 weak abilities. Any lower score calls into question the organization's ability to survive (Van Doren and Smith, 1985).

This self-study facilitates the commitment by the administration to include marketing as an integral part of the organization's planning process. If the investment of marketing is to be successful, commitment must be present.

STAFF COMMITMENT

Once the administrator and board have committed to the agency's involvement in marketing, it is essential to involve the staff in the planning process as much as possible. For all the staff to be committed and supportive, they must understand the rationale, purposes, goals, objectives, strategies, and tactics of marketing (Alward, 1983).

Many professional staff members view marketing as something negative or feel that the marketing person should do it. Too often staff members view marketing as simply promotional efforts in which they play no part. Also, members may feel that they lack marketing skills and thus choose not to participate in marketing efforts.

To gain the acceptance of marketing with the staff, it must be explained that marketing is finding out what people want and giving

Table 4.1 Nonprofit Marketing Analysis for Organizational Self-Study

Rank the organization from 5 (high) to 1 (low).

Orientation

The organization:

1. Is aware of clients' needs, problems, and opportunities. _____
2. Is aware of contributors' needs, problems, and opportunities. _____
3. Uses rational and emotional appeals to present benefits to clients and contributors. _____
4. Has knowledge of products and services so facts can be used to support promised benefits. _____
5. Knows its competition for clients and contributors. _____
6. Has developed a unique approach of distinguishing benefit from that of competition. _____
7. Targets or directs marketing efforts to a defined group of clients or contributors. _____

Research

The organization:

8. Plans and conducts research to learn about clients' and contributors' needs, problems, and opportunities. _____
9. Analyzes and uses research to adjust offerings to clients' and contributors' needs, problems, and opportunities. _____
10. Has designated individuals responsible for ongoing research. _____

Marketing Planning

The organization:

11. Concentrates on long-term planning versus detailed how-to lists. _____
12. Develops a 3-year marketing plan for the organizaiton. _____
13. Has several strategies for marketing products or services to each target market of clients and contributors. _____
14. Includes products and services, price, place, and promotion in planning its marketing efforts. _____
15. Fully markets, rather than simply promotes, its products. _____
16. Has designated individuals responsible for implementing major marketing strategies. _____

Table 4.1   (*Continued*)

17. Has fixed a time line for major marketing strategies. _____

Marketing Control

The organization:

18. Uses evaluation measures to assess implementation of the plan. _____
19. Uses the feedback to redirect the orientation, research, and marketing planning of the group. _____
20. Has a person designated as the head marketer. _____

Source: Van Doren, D., Smith, L. Self-analysis can gauge marketing orientation. *Marketing News,* 19 (25)(December 6, 1985):14. Reprinted from *Marketing News,* published by the American Marketing Association.

them more of it. All nurses, social workers, physical therapists, and other health professionals have been taught in their educational programs to assess the need of the client and then develop a plan of care. Marketing uses the same process. By having staff input on the needs they see that clients have, they can help the agency determine what services will be needed to develop a plan of care for those clients.

It is also the responsibility of each staff member to show the client how he or she can best meet the client's needs. Staff members may not think it's their job to sell the agency's services, but simply by being employees of that agency staff members communicate an image. What image the client gets depends on the staff member. Understanding what the agency is trying to do, the services it offers, how it is managed, and whether it complies with standards, helps a staff member articulate an image to the client. For staff to market the services and to be committed, it is important for them to understand the big picture of the agency. This especially is true when agencies hire a lot of contract employees. These staff members need a good orientation to the marketing philosophy and strategy of the agency so that they can market the agency appropriately.

The other aspect of commitment of staff to marketing is to build on the strengths of the staff member's and have them carry out roles appropriate to these strengths.

Hanks (1982) describes various skills people have and how to combine them to create a good team. The administrator or marketing manager has to look for these skills in the staff and bring them together to develop a marketing team. Having people do what they are good at enhances commitment to the project or plan because staff members are being recognized for their skills. The skills Hanks (1982: 139) describes are

Creator: originates ideas

Developer: develops ideas

Implementor: puts developed ideas into real-world context

Seller: sells ideas to others

Maintainer: keeps management or production of an idea going

Evaluator: judges how well results match purpose

Solver: locates and defines problems and proposes solutions

All these skills are necessary to implement a marketing plan. The plan must be based on the agency's staff and the skills they possess. Everyone does not have to have the same commitment, but a balance can be reached by using the strengths of the staff.

BUDGET ALLOCATION

Not only is a commitment needed, but resources must be allocated for development of a market plan. Hauser (1984: 75) has commented that "nothing makes an agency's degree of commitment to marketing clearer than its marketing budget." The banking industry, which many compare to the health care industry, has used a formula of $1,000 for every $1 million of deposits as the amount a bank should put into its marketing budget. As competition has increased the formula has changed to a flat 1%–2% of an organization's overall operating budget. In a survey conducted by Byrne Associates (1986) of 455 home health care agencies in August 1986, agency's were asked what percentage of their budget they directed toward marketing. Two thirds of the 73 respondents indicated that they had a marketing budget. The average for those with marketing budgets was 1.7% of the agency budget. The marketing budget was used to pay for market planning, audits, market research, design, graphics, public relations, and advertising. However, expenditure of money does not alone guarantee the success of marketing.

RESOURCE ALLOCATION

Money is not the only resource that must be allocated in order to develop a market plan. The checklist shown in Figure 4.1 shows some of the other resources that must be considered.

If some of the resources are not available, the agency must determine whether resources can be diverted to developing a market plan or whether they can be acquired. For example, if an agency lacks knowledge about how to do market research, it could contact a university in the area with a marketing class and invite its professor and students to conduct an actual survey at the agency.

If there is commitment but not availability of resources or a plan to divert resources for marketing, a market plan cannot be developed. A successful market plan cannot be developed if there is commitment without resources or resources without commitment. If an investment is made wisely in the beginning to commit to market planning, the agency will better be able to optimize its abilities.

☐ Personnel
☐ Money
☐ Equipment
☐ Space
☐ Time
☐ Knowledge
☐ Data or information
☐ Internal political influence or power

Figure 4.1. Checklist of resources.

CONCLUSION

For a market plan to be successful, commitment from the administration and staff is essential. If commitment is lacking, the plan will not be utilized or accepted.

The commitment of the administration can be assessed by using a self-study tool. Questions are asked about the orientation of the organization, the role of research in the organization, the amount of marketing planning, and the type of market control. Scores are then given that rate the agency in marketing. This tool helps the administration focus on where their weaknesses are.

Commitment of the staff is also important. For staff to be supportive, they must understand the rationale, purpose, goals, objectives, strategies, and tactics of marketing. Building a marketing team means drawing on the strengths of the staff so they will feel committed to the plan.

Budget and resource allocation needs to be assessed as the market plan is started. If adequate resources are not available initially, it will be very difficult to develop a worthwhile product.

REFERENCES

Alward, R. A marketing approach to nursing administration, part 2. *Journal of Nursing Administration.* (April 1983):18–21.

Byrne Associates. *Marketing and Management Survey.* St. Louis: Byrne Associates, August 1986.

Hanks, K. *Motivating People.* Allen, TX: Argus Communications, 1982.

Hauser, L. 10 reasons hospital marketing programs fail. *Hospitals.* (September 1984): 75.

Ireland, R. Using marketing strategies to put hospitals on target. *Journal of American Hospital Association.* 51(June 1, 1977):54–57.

Van Doren, D., Smith, L. Self-analysis can gauge marketing orientation. *Marketing News.* (December 6, 1985):14. Vol. 19, No. 25.

Walter C. Academic medical center features image analysis in marketing audit. *Hospitals.* (August 16, 1981):92. Vol. 10, No. 16.

5

Market Audit

Agencies must take a critical look at themselves and their marketing performance. Marketing is an area that requires consistent monitoring of plans and interventions. One method of analysis of the agency's marketing strategy is to conduct a marketing audit. The audit not only reviews the past but also speculates about changes that will affect the agency and its search for new markets.

A marketing audit is defined as a "comprehensive, systematic, independent, and periodic examination of an organization's marketing environment, objectives, strategies, and activities with a view of determining problem areas and opportunities and recommending a plan of action to improve the organization's marketing performance" (Kotler et al., 1977: 27). A marketing audit has the following characteristics (Kotler, 1982):

1. Comprehensive: covers all major marketing issues, not just trouble spots, facing the organization
2. Systematic: involves an orderly process of diagnostic steps defining the organization's internal and external environment and specific marketing activities, the diagnosis is followed by a corrective action plan to improve the organization's overall marketing effectiveness
3. Independent: conducted by an inside or outside individual who can gain management's confidence and has the needed objectivity
4. Periodic: carried out periodically, rather than when there is a crisis

A variety of reasons exist for conducting a marketing audit. The dynamic nature of our health care system requires an organization to have up-to-date information. The benefits a home health care agency receives from a marketing audit are that it (1) may identify or anticipate problems associated with the organization's marketing activities; (2) may uncover marketing opportunities that could be pursued or additional target markets that could be cultivated; (3) should help establish marketing goals and effective marketing strategies for reaching those goals; and (4) may suggest new or different ways of organizing and implementing marketing activities (Schlinger, 1985).

The audit should be carried out by one or more staff members or outside consultants. If staff are used, caution must be taken in the selection of the staff members to assure that they can be objective. It is important that such individuals do not assume they know the information but search for data both inside and outside the agency.

Table 5.1 is a guide to the kinds of questions that the marketing auditor needs to investigate. Completing this audit will involve participation from many different staff members. Parts of the audit could be assigned to various staff members, and the auditor could bring it all together. Some agencies have found an audit committee the most workable situation. Whatever the model, involving the staff enables all members to feel they have contributed to the planning and future of the agency.

MARKET AND MARKET SEGMENTS

To begin the market audit, it is necessary to define the market geographically, demographically, and numerically. The market for the agency may be all of a city and county, with a focus on the elderly population that is ill and needs skilled nursing care. Other markets could be the acute pediatric client, the well adult, or the female maternity client. Each of these markets is examined with regard to the following variables:

Geographic   Nation, state, region, city, county, neighborhood

Demographic   Age, sex, family size, marital status, life-style, income, occupation, education, religion, race

Numerical   Potential users, users, ex-users, usage pattern of users, service usage, loyalty to agency, readiness for services, attitude toward services

An example of a market segment profile for an elderly population is

1. Widowed, living alone, good health, active, affluent
2. Widowed, living alone, good health, inactive, affluent
3. Widowed, nursing home, poor health, inactive
4. Living with spouse, good health, active, moderate income
5. Widowed, retirement home, fair health, inactive, moderate income
6. Widowed, living with children, fair health, active, moderate income (Ireland, 1986)

Table 5.1 Market Audit Questions

Market and Market Segments

1. Describe your market geographically.
2. How is your market grouped?
3. How do the following factors affect your market?

   Age of population

   Income of population

   Occupation

   Demographic shifts

   Geographic trends

   Seasons of the year

   Other
4. How many potential clients do you have?
5. How many of them are aware of your organization's services?

Organization

1. What is the basic philosophy of your organization?
2. What are the goals and objectives of your organization?
3. What are your organization's strengths and weaknesses? (See Worksheet A.)
4. Where has your organization's growth come from?
5. Where do you expect the growth to come from in the future?
6. How do conditions in other industries affect your organization?
7. What internal controls affect your organization?

   Advisory board

   Stockholders

   Board of directors

   Staff
8. What external controls affect your organization?

   Local

   State

   Federal

   Self-regulation
9. What regulatory or legislative trends will affect your organization?

(Continued)

WORKSHEET A
STRENGTHS AND WEAKNESSES

Item	Strengths	Weaknesses
Management		
Financial resources		
Staffing		
Facilities and equipment		
Services		
Image		
Reputation		
Other		

Table 5.1 (*Continued*)

Client

1. What is the profile of present or potential users of your service?
2. How is your client profile different from that of the competition?
3. What is the frequency and quantity of client usage of your service?
4. Why do clients purchase or utilize your services?
5. Who makes the buying or utilization decision?

Competitors

1. How many competitors do you have?
2. Is this number decreasing or increasing?
3. Who are your principal competitors? (See Worksheet B.)
4. What is your competitors' share of the marketplace?
5. Is competition on a price or nonprice basis? (See Worksheet C.)
6. Where does the competition seem to be heading?

Services and Products

1. Analyze your services and products. (See Worksheet D.)
2. Are there any voids?
3. Do you plan to address these voids? How?

Pricing

1. What is the pricing philosophy of your organization?
2. How are the prices for services determined?
3. How do your prices compare with those of the competition?
4. How is your pricing viewed by

   Clients

   Decision makers

   Third-party payers

   Organizations

   Other

Promotion and Advertising

1. What is the objective of the organization's present promotional and advertising material?

(Continued)

WORKSHEET B
COMPETITOR DATA

Organization name _____

Address _____

_____

Branch offices _____

Number of staff _____ Major clients _____

_____

Reputation and image _____

_____

Key personnel

Name _____		_____
Title _____		_____
Background _____		_____
Strengths _____		_____
_____		_____
Weaknesses _____		_____

Pricing policies _____

_____

Marketing and promotional activities _____

_____

_____

_____

_____

_____

_____

WORKSHEET C
COMPETITOR ANALYSIS

List each feature or attribute of your agency and those of your competitors. Rate the the strength of each feature or attribute on a scale of 0 to 5 (0, lowest; 5, highest). Total each column to determine relative competitive strength or identify areas of potential vulnerability.

Feature or Attribute	Your Firm	Competitor 1	Competitor 2	Competitor 3	Competitor 4
24-hour nursing	5	1	0	2	5
Occupational therapy	4	3	4	1	5
Physical therapy	3	3	4	3	4
Homemakers	3	0	5	3	5
Trained staff	4	3	4	4	5
Medicare	5	5	0	5	0
Direct pay	2	1	5	1	5
Total	26	16	22	20	29

WORKSHEET D
SERVICE AND PRODUCT ANALYSIS

Service or Product	Distinctive Features	Benefit to Client	How Viewed by Client	Total Cost	↑ or ↓	Why Heavily Utilized or Not

Table 5.1   *(Continued)*

2. How does promotional and advertising material support your marketing objectives?

3. What materials and activities will you use to create and maintain your image?

4. How are these materials and activities evaluated for results?

5. How are promotional materials and advertising integrated into personal selling?

Place

1. Where are you located in relation to your clients?

2. When did you last evaluate your present location?

3. What suppliers do you deal with?

4. What materials do you need on hand?

An example for a well adult is

1. Single, living alone, city resident, good health, active, lower middle class, 20–30 years old

2. Single, living alone, city resident, good health, inactive, upper middle class, 30–40 years old

3. Married, living with spouse, city resident, good health, inactive, upper middle class, 25–35 years old

4. Divorced, living alone, county resident, good health, active, lower middle class, 30–35 years old

From these data the agency can determine the best potential target for its services. If the home health care agency is going to start health and fitness talks, which market segment would be the best initial target?

On a larger scale of market segmentation, the United States General Accounting Office conducted a survey of Medicare use in home health care. They segmented the market into five types of home health care users. Table 5.2 demonstrates how home health care users nationwide can be segmented.

In numerical terms, the agency must examine how many users it currently has, the usage pattern of those users (e.g., once a week or once a month), and what services are being utilized (e.g., nursing, physical therapy, occupational therapy, or social work).

It is also important to know how many potential clients the agency has and how many of them are aware of the organization. This can be done by using census data to determine how many people live in the city or area the agency serves. Telephone surveys have been found to be an effective way of determining how many clients know about an agency's services. Legg and Lamb (1986) found in a random sample telephone survey that only 13% of the respondents could identify one or more specific activity or program provided by the agency. Thus, public awareness was very low.

Another factor to consider is the loyalty of users to the agency. Clients should be asked whether they would use your agency a second time, refer their friends to you, and request your agency when they are in the hospital?

Often agencies spend time simply educating all age groups to what home care is. Prospective clients may not need home care today, but they may remember your services and your agency when they are ready for home care, or they may tell a friend who needs home care about your services and your agency. Readiness can be evaluated by assessing whether prospective clients are unaware, aware, informed, interested, intending to use, or are using.

Combined with readiness is the attitude people or users display about the service. Are they enthusiastic, positive, negative, disinterested, or indifferent?

These are the attitudes the agency can assess in potential and actual users of their services. Once the attitudes are identified the agency can develop methods of changing negative or indifferent attitudes and supporting enthusiastic or positive attitudes.

By determining and describing the market and market segmentation, the agency can better plan how to promote its services so that the information reaches the intended audience.

THE ORGANIZATION

The second step in the audit is to determine the organization's philosophy, goals, objectives, strengths, weaknesses, and possibilities for growth. The basic philosophy of the organization is a statement of beliefs that directs one's practice and is a framework for all plans and activities.

Table 5.2 Profiles of Types of Home Health Care Users

Type I (25.4%)	Type II (20.9%)	Type III (24.4%)	Type IV (15.3%)	Type V (13.9%)
		Medical Condition		
Absence of problem in 20 of 29 medical conditions[a]	Absence of problem in 16 of 29 medical conditions	Absence of problem in 20 of 29 medical conditions	Absence of problem in 10 of 29 medical conditions	Absence of problem in 9 of 29 medical conditions
	Distinguishing conditions: broken hip, other broken bones, glaucoma, rheumatism	Distinguishing conditions: cancer, glaucoma	Distinguishing conditions: heart attack, other heart problems, bronchitis, flu, asthma, rheumatism, permanent stiffness, glaucoma, diabetes, constipation, insomnia, obesity, arteriosclerosis, circulatory problems, pneumonia, emphysema	Distinguishing conditions: paralysis, multiple sclerosis, cerebral palsy, Parkinson's disease, mental retardation, senility, stroke, permanent stiffness, constipation, arteriosclerosis, circulatory problems

Activities of Daily Living

Absence of problem	Getting in and out of bed, getting around house, bathing, using the toilet	Getting in and out of bed, getting around house, bathing, dressing, using the toilet	Bathing	Assistance needed in all 6 activities of daily living

Instrumental Activities of Daily Living

Absence of problem in 8 of 10 activities[b]	Heavy housework, grocery shopping, transportation, getting around outside	Assistance needed in all 10 activities	Assistance needed in 8 of 10 activities	Assistance needed in all 10 activities

Other

			Bedfast, wheelchair fast, unable to do inside activities

---

[a]Although type I was not distinguished by specific medical conditions, the following conditions were present within the type: rheumatism, diabetes cancer, insomnia, obesity, hypertension, circulatory problems, pneumonia, and emphysema.

[b]Although type I was not distinguished by specific instrumental activities of daily living, this group had limitations in heavy housework and laundry.

Source: United States General Accounting Office. *Medicare: Need to Strengthen Home Health Care Payment Controls and Address Unmet Needs.* Publicaiton no. HRD-87-9. Washington, DC: Government Printing Office, 1986, 24.

Cardinal Ritter Institute Home Care Program in St. Louis summarizes their philosophy in their brochure:

There's no place like home. . . . We believe that and we know you do too. Friendly faces, familiar things, the special warmth you find just inside your own front door—there's no substitute for that kind of medicine.

This is the reason the Cardinal Ritter Institute has a Home Health Care Program . . . to provide health care to persons in their own homes. This service is directed toward the whole person and is implemented through the cooperative efforts of a fully qualified health team.

—Cardinal Ritter Institute, 1986

From reading this philosophy, conclusions can be drawn about the services the institute offers and why it offers them. The marketing plan is then developed to help carry out the agency's mission.

The process of philosophy development can be enlightening in itself. Often it will be found that there is no consensus about an organization's philosophy. Answers to questions about what business an agency is in and its basic purpose may vary greatly. Consensus must be reached before further steps are taken to work on goals and objectives.

From the philosophy, goals and objectives are identified. An example from the philosophy of the Cardinal Ritter Institute is its goal to help older people and their families meet the challenges and difficulties of growing older (Cardinal Ritter Institute, 1986). Objectives address providing home health care services, making apartments available to the elderly, providing a comprehensive range of social services, and coordinating volunteers who want to help others.

From the philosophy, the organization's strengths and weaknesses are identified. In Table 5.1, Worksheet A can help the agency to examine the seven major components of its organization: (1) management, (2) financial resources, (3) staffing, (4) facilities and equipment, (5) services, (6) image, and (7) reputation.

Each of these components must be critically and objectively evaluated. For example, an assessment of an agency may determine a strength to be over 25 years of experience in home health care, but a weakness may be that staff members are not skilled in the new technology needed for some clients. Another audit of the agency may determine that management is weak because of lack of health care experience. Determining strengths and weaknesses is a good activity to involve the entire staff in because perception of management, staff, and clients may be very different. Input is needed from all areas.

To look toward the future the agency examines where it expects growth to come from in the future. Will it be in the acute pediatric care area or in visiting new mothers. In examining all these factors, the internal and external controls of the organization must be considered. Controls include boards of directors, federal regulations, and legislations. It is imperative that the agency actively participate in state and national home care associations to keep updated on these controls as well as to help inform the decision makers on how their regulations and laws will affect home health care.

THE CLIENT

The third step in the market audit is to develop a profile of the agency's clients. Are the clients elderly, on Medicare, and in need of skilled nursing care or are they high-risk infants who need monitoring for growth and development? It is also important to determine whether an agency's client profile is different from that of the competition. From reading various agency brochures, it can be determined whether an agency's clients are elderly, pediatric, or terminally ill and whether they require rehabilitative services, skilled nursing care, or personal care. Some agency's specialize, offering, for example, only care for the terminally ill patient. Be aware of the client profile of the competition.

Other factors to consider regarding the client are the frequency and quantity of client usage of the service. This can be summarized from records kept at the agency for reimbursement. This knowledge helps to identify the pattern of usage.

Why clients purchase or utilize your services is very important to determine. The answers to these questions can determine the benefits the agency offers the public and should be conveyed to the public through the agency's promotional material. It is important to conduct client surveys or interviews periodically or at the close of a client's record in order to obtain the client's feedback about the services. Table 5.3 shows an example of one such survey.

The last piece of client information is who makes the buying decision regarding home care. In examining the *Missouri Profile of Home Health Agencies*, the physician is the predominant referral agent. Legg and Lamb (1986) also found that the physician seeks information from nurses or social service workers before making

Table 5.3   Tell Us What You Think

Thank you for allowing us to serve you during your recent admission to our home health care agency. We work very hard to make every patient's experience with our agency positive and continually try to make our services better. Your evaluation of the services you received will help us make any necessary improvements.

1. Were staff members courteous in their telephone contact with you?
   Yes ( )   No ( )
   Comments:

2. How would you rate the attitude of agency personnel involved with your care?

	Excellent	Good	Fair	Poor	Did Not Use
Home health nurse	( )	( )	( )	( )	( )
Physical therapist	( )	( )	( )	( )	( )
Occupational therapist	( )	( )	( )	( )	( )
Speech therapist	( )	( )	( )	( )	( )
Social worker	( )	( )	( )	( )	( )
Home health aide	( )	( )	( )	( )	( )
Homemaker	( )	( )	( )	( )	( )

3. How would you rate the quality of care you received from agency involved with your care?

	Excellent	Good	Fair	Poor	Did Not Use
Home health nurse	( )	( )	( )	( )	( )
Physical therapist	( )	( )	( )	( )	( )
Occuaptional therapist	( )	( )	( )	( )	( )
Speech therapist	( )	( )	( )	( )	( )
Social worker	( )	( )	( )	( )	( )
Home health aide	( )	( )	( )	( )	( )
Homemaker	( )	( )	( )	( )	( )

4. Did you feel confident of the ability of the person rendering the service?
   Yes ( )   No ( )
   Comments:

5. Were your or your family taught how to continue necessary care when the agency services were discontinued?
Yes ( )   No ( )
Comments:

6. Were financial arrangements handled in a satisfactory manner?
Yes ( )   No ( )
Comments:

7. Was the service you received carried out to your expectations?
Yes ( )   No ( )
Comments:

8. Would you recommend our agency to anyone else?
Yes ( )   No ( )
Comments:

9. Would you contact our agency if you needed home care again?
Yes ( )   No ( )
Comments:

10. If there is anything you would change about our agency what would it be?

referrals for home health services or delegates referral responsibility to those parties. The consumer or family has been low on the list of those who influence the buying decision. With the growing consumer movement, this fact may change greatly in the future. Consumers can also put pressure on physicians or social workers to request the home health agency they want to use.

COMPETITORS

The analysis of competitors is becoming critical as the home health care market becomes increasingly competitive. Marketers should regularly and systematically utilize numerous sources for competitive evaluations. Sources of data would include

- Trade shows
- Trade associations
- Government publications
- Durable medical companies
- Physicians and discharge planners
- Trade magazines
- Local health officials
- Related business contacts, advertising agencies, bankers, lawyers, accountants, and consultants
- Professional service and social clubs or associations
- Previous employees of competitors
- Telephone and association directories
- Agency's own employees
- State statistical reports
- Advertising campaigns
- Manuals and brochures

From these sources, the agency can identify how many competitors it has and whether this number is increasing or decreasing. It is important to record this information and keep it on file. Table 5.1, Worksheet B is a competitor data sheet that is used to obtain data on the competition. If such a sheet is on file, it is available to the entire staff, not just kept in someone's head.

It is also important to determine the competitor's share of the marketplace. This information can be obtained from the input of discharge planners, physicians, and clients as to what services they are using currently. Listening to sources previously identified will also help an agency consider or predict where a competitor may be reading.

In developing these profiles and information, data can be summarized using a tool such as Table 5.1, Worksheet C. This analysis will allow the agency to determine areas where it might strengthen its services. Each competitive agency is scored on the relative strength of given features. Scores are then totaled, and major competitors can be identified. This analysis sheet also shows how well your agency compares to others. Identifying where your agency's competitors have higher scores may mean that adjustments must be made to improve your agency's services.

SERVICES AND PRODUCTS

Next the agency should examine the services and products it delivers. One of the first questions that can be asked is whether the services that the agency offers match the philosophy of the agency. Table 5.1, Worksheet D illustrates a service and product analysis to determine what benefit clients receive and how well each service is utilized. These data are collected from staff, interviews with clients and outside agency personnel, questionnaires, and agency financial information. The first column simply states the service or product, such as skilled nursing care. Then the distinctive features of that service or product are explained. Features are facts about a service or product that are present in its design. For example, features include intravenous therapy services and 24-hour-a-day registered nurse coverage. From this information, the benefits to the client are determined. A benefit is an advantage to the client because of the feature. Here you can ask yourself, "Just because we have skilled nursing care for 24-hour coverage, what benefit does this give the client?" Examples of benefits are peace of mind from knowing that care can be given whenever it is needed and the fact that there is someone the client can rely upon for assistance.

It is helpful at this point to validate with the client how they view the services or products the agency offers. Interviews, short telephone follow-ups, or questionnaires can be used to determine the client's opinion of the services or products.

The total cost of the service or product is detailed, as is the charge to the client. This information enables the agency to identify high-cost services and products as well as high-profit areas. From these data, the agency predicts whether various services or products should be increased or decreased.

The agency then needs to question why a service or product is heavily utilized or why it is not? Maybe the major source of referrals or referral agents view your agency as the best at providing that specialized service.

When the analysis is filled out, it should be examined for voids. If voids are found, the agency must address whether it plans to do something about the void and, if so, what that course of action should be.

PRICING

Pricing is closely related to specific services and products. The pricing philosophy of the agency must first be explored. Is it a tax-supported or United Way agency, or is it profit making? Does the agency accept Medicare and Medicaid for reimbursement or only private insurance and direct pay. The answers to these questions will reflect the philosophy of the agency and will influence pricing. In determining prices, home health care agencies differ from manufacturers and other service agencies. In many of these businesses the price is set by the cost to the business, percent profit, and what the market will bear; these businesses are not dependent on reimbursement as payment for their products or services. Home health care pricing is largely driven by the reimbursement system. In the future, much of the pricing may be determined by a diagnosis-related group (DRG) system for home care, in which there is a set reimbursement for the client's diagnosis. Fees set by the agency must be compared with those of the competition to see if they are indeed competitive.

Besides the dollar amount of prices, the client faces other costs. These costs are sometimes termed the social costs and include the expenditure of time and effort, the potential effect on the client's life-style, and the psychic risk to the client's pride or sense of control. Such costs can also include the family's efforts to arrange home health services, their worry about whether caretakers will be there when they are supposed to, and their concern about whether they are doing the right thing for their loved one. These costs are not easy to evaluate in terms of dollars and cents.

The other aspect of pricing is how the fees will be viewed by clients, decision makers, third-party payers, organizations, and other agencies. The agency may set a fee and find that clients perceive the care to be of lower quality because of a lower price. Pricing above a reimbursable rate requires the agency to devote more time to fee collection.

PROMOTION AND ADVERTISING

In the area of promotion and advertising, the agency must first decide the objective it wants to achieve. Is the promotional objective to increase the public's awareness of the agency's services, or is it to increase client usage of the services by 5%? These are two different objectives and involve different promotional and advertising strategies. Once the objective is determined, the agency needs to question how to present advertising material that supports the objective. If the current material does not support the objective or additional material is needed, then the agency must describe the materials needed.

Agencies use brochures, public service announcements, direct mailing, workshops, personal selling, and paid advertisements to communicate with the client. The type of material developed depends to a large extent on the financial resources of the agency. Creating material at the agency rather than having it done by outside advertising agencies reduces costs but may not result in a high-quality product. Detailed descriptions of promotion and promotional activities in which an agency can participate are discussed in Chapter 9.

It is important not only to use the promotional material but to evaluate its effectiveness. If direct mailing is used, you should follow up with people to see if they have questions about your services. Asking someone how they heard of your agency is another simple method. Further methods of evaluation are discussed in Chapter 8.

PLACE

The last part of the audit is to examine whether your agency is situated in a location convenient to your client. Many agencies do not have to worry about clients coming to them, but they do need to think about nurses coming into the agency for charting or reporting and also being in close proximity to the agency's major referral sources. It is also important to consider whether the agency serves a wide geographic area and whether all the services are centralized in one area or the agency has outreach offices in other locations.

The agency should conduct a periodic evaluation of the distribution of the services and the office locations. Many home health care agencies find it very costly to manage outreach offices that do not produce a high volume of cases. Such agencies pull back to a centralized location and subcontract work in outreach areas.

Not only is office location considered in price, but so are the supplies the agency needs on hand and how the agency will deal with suppliers. Many home health agencies have solved this problem by establishing a profit arm and setting up a durable medical equipment company. Others have contracts with specific companies to service the clients of the agency. Adding equipment companies and contracting with specific companies can promote more comprehensive, dependable service for the client.

After the completion of the market audit, the agency has an in-depth analysis of its organization. From this analysis, future directions for the agency can be determined.

CONCLUSION

Agencies must take a critical look at themselves and their marketing performance. A market audit is a way of examining the agency's marketing strategy.

Marketing audits need to be comprehensive, systematic, independent, and periodic. A variety of means exist for conducting a market audit, and various people may conduct an audit. Staff members or outside consultants can be used, but it is important that the individuals are objective and that they explore for data.

An audit is usually composed of questions addressed to the agency regarding the following areas: market and market segments, organization, clients, competitors, products and services, pricing, promotion and advertising, and place. By answering questions regarding all these areas of operation, an agency can identify problem or opportunity areas that should be explored. This method of auditing helps to prepare an agency to meet the challenges of a rapidly changing market.

REFERENCES

Cardinal Ritter Institute. Home care program brochure. St. Louis: 1986.

Ireland, R. Marketing for Home Care. Conference of the Missouri Association of Home Health Agencies. Kansas City, MO: December 9, 1986.

Kotler, P. *Marketing for Non-Profit Organizations* (2d ed.). Englewood Cliffs, NJ: Prentice-Hall, 1982.

Kotler, P., Gregor, W., Rodgers, W. The marketing audit comes of age. *Sloan Management Review.* 8(Winter 1977):25–43.

Legg, D., Lamb, C. The role of referral agencies in the Marketing of home health services. *Journal of Health Care Marketing.* 6(March 1986):51–56.

Missouri Department of Health. *Missouri Profile of Home Health Agencies.* Jefferson City, Missouri, 1986.

Schlinger, M. J. Marketing audits for health organizations: a practical guide in *Health Care Marketing Issues and Trends.* Cooper, P. (ed.). Rockville, MD: Aspen, 1985, 136–149.

United States General Accounting Office. *Medicare: Need to Strengthen Home Health Care Payment Controls and Address Unmet Needs.* Publication no. HRD-87-9. Washington, DC: Government Printing Office, 1986.

6

*Planning
Phase*

Problem identification is meaningless without action toward a solution. Such action is initiated through planning. Planning implies a decision-making process directed at introducing change (Braden, 1976).

Friedman (1967) describes planning as a guidance of change within a system. As a self-guidance system, planning (1) confronts the expected with intended performance, (2) sets up controls to accomplish the intended, (3) observes variance from intended paths of change, and (4) initiates a new cycle to cope with significant variations from the intended.

PLANNING MODELS

Planning to produce a change offers hope for a reasonable and peaceful means of defining, securing agreement on, and introducing change. As an agency begins the planning process, it must identify the framework it will use to plan.

Every agency must assess what it believes about planning. Is methodical planning strongly emphasized, or is crisis planning the mode of the agency? The attitudes of agency personnel will influence the planning mode that will be accepted. Possible planning modes are laissez-faire, disjointed incrementalism, allocative, problem solving, exploitive, explorative, normative, and total planning (Blum, 1974). Table 6.1 illustrates the differences among these planning models. If the agency has a tendency to react to existing conditions rather than to change them, it would be likely to accept a laissez-faire, disjointed incrementalism, or allocative planning approach. If the agency is a trend setter and wants to control where the home health industry will go, it would be likely use an exploitive or explorative mode.

The different planning modes simply set the framework of how planning will be done within the agency and the role the agency will play in the health care arena. For example, let us contrast an agency that selects the laissez-faire mode with one that chooses the exploitive mode. Let us assume that it is predicted that reimbursed home health services under Medicare will be decreased. Agencies are already seeing an increase in the number of denials, and the agencies are worried because over 50% of their revenue comes from Medicare.

The laissez-faire agency would simply be worried about the changes and the current situation. Its hope is that the regulations will not be passed and therefore the reimbursable services will at least remain

Table 6.1 Planning Models

Characteristics	Laissez-Faire	Disjointed Incrementalism	Allocative	Problem Solving	Exploitive	Explorative	Normative	Total Planning
Planning approach	No planning, competitive market provides consumer choice	Minimal planning to remedy undesirable solutions when they become intolerable	Minimal planning to balance allocation of resources for future	Plan for present or near future by analyzing problems, developing interventions, and allocating resources	Plan for future by making the most of trends and allocating resources	Plan for future and design feasible future	Plan for future by deciding on desired future and allocating resources to that trend	Plan for present and future by deciding specific goals for desired future
Short-term results	Problems will disappear	Lessen present problems	Alter priorities and present problems	Lessen present problems	Take advantage of what is coming	Choose feasible destiny	Help create destiny	Control all destiny
Long-term results	Future will be what it is to be	Modify future by reducing present problems	Balance and modify future by avoiding obvious problems	Improve future by reducing problems	Unbalance and modify future	Modify future by aiming for what could be	Modify future by aiming for what ought to be	Modify future by aiming for what policy makers or planners have said will be
Direction of intervention	No direct intervention	Alter system only	Leave system alone, optimize resources	Modify system and environment to control problems	Modify system to get what is wanted	Improve old system or fashion new one	Change system as consistent with goals	Force actions to fit proposed system
Nature of participation	None	Involve those who show up	Involve groups in power	Involve groups relevant to the issue	Involve groups in power	Involve all relevant participants of society	Involve all relevant participants of society	Involve planners, technologists, and those in power
Time to obtain desired effects	Not relevant	Fast	Fast	Moderately prompt	Slow	Very slow	Very slow	Moderately prompt
Cost to obtain desired effects	Not relevant	Modest	Low	Modest	Low	High	High	Very high

Source: Blum, H. *Planning for Health*. New York: Human Sciences Press, 1974, 56–59.

the same. This agency decides that there is nothing it can do to influence this decision by the government, so it decides not to try. The administration also decides not to tell staff members about this possible problem because it does not want the staff to think the agency has a financial problem.

In contrast, the exploitive model agency decides that it needs to plan ways to address the possibility of decreased reimbursement. It develops strategies for contacting legislators, Health Care Financing Administration personnel, consumers, and retired persons' groups. All staff members are asked to participate and are assigned people to contact about the impact of decreased reimbursement on the home care patient population. The administration also realizes that it cannot continue to depend so heavily on Medicare reimbursement and decides to conduct a detailed marketing study of potential markets to diversify their revenues. Staff and managers are asked to participate in this project, which is directed and coordinated by the marketing manager.

The laissez-faire agency lets the future take its own course, while the exploitive agency tries to modify the system and make the most of trends. All agencies have to decide which mode they are comfortable with and then plan accordingly.

Table 6.2 is an example of a planning worksheet that can be used in organizing a plan to address a problem that has been identified. This worksheet will be used to demonstrate the process of identifying a problem and developing strategies to arrive at an appropriate solution.

PROBLEM IDENTIFICATION

As the process begins to reveal problems or opportunities from the marketing audit, the planner must decide which of four marketing strategies to implement. These strategies are market penetration, market development, product development, and diversification (Rubright and MacDonald, 1981).

The market penetration strategy is aimed at getting the agency a bigger share of the business in its current arena of operation. Market development strategies are designed to find new targets to serve in the present service area or to expand that area to include new targets. Product development calls for changing or improving an organization's services and effectiveness. The purpose of diversification is to find completely new kinds of services or programs to offer to a target

TABLE 6.2
PLANNING WORKSHEET

Problem: _____

_____

_____

Goal: _____

_____

Objectives: _____

_____

_____

_____

_____

Strategy ideas:

Strategy 1	Strategy 2	Strategy 3

Selected Strategy: _____

_____

_____

market. As the market audit is examined, these marketing strategies should serve as a guide as to which marketing plans should be implemented.

The following questions can help the marketer determine problem and opportunity areas for the agency:

1. What has changed?
    Market
    Organization
    Client
    Competitors
    Products and services
    Pricing
    Promotion and advertising
    Place
2. Where are the discrepancies?
3. Where are the weaknesses?
4. Where are the strengths?
5. What resources are not being utilized?
6. What standards are not being met?
7. What are the values of the client?
8. What are the unmet needs of clients?
9. What conditions can something be done about?
10. Where are the priorities of the agency?

Answers to these questions will allow the agency to identify a problem list from which strategies are developed.

Changes

In examining change, the agency looks for trends that are occurring. Regardless of whether the trends are good or bad, they influence the agency and the services offered. Each component of the marketing audit needs to be analyzed to determine whether change has occurred or will occur and how that change has influenced or will influence services. For example, if population statistics show that in 2 years the largest population group will be the "older old" (75 years and up), this means that services directed toward care, rather than preventive services, will be in greater demand. Then the agency must examine whether it has such services in place or what it must do to prepare for this change.

Discrepancies

Discrepancies are differences or disagreements between statements. As the audit is done, the marketer must continually cross-reference what the data report. If the agency's literature says it offers 24-hour services but staffing patterns indicate a problem in finding nurses to work night shifts, there is a discrepancy. This discrepancy needs to be examined and a solution to the problem found.

Weaknesses

Weaknesses are usually areas where something is inadequate or where there is a flaw or a shortcoming. For example, in examining the financial aspects of the organization, the lag between submitting insurance and getting paid may cause a cash flow problem for the agency. This flow needs to be examined further to find a solution.

Strengths

Areas of the agency that are effective and are producing well are strengths for that agency. These are the areas that the business needs to enhance and use to resolve some of the identified problems. Strengths can include good management, adequate capital, longevity of staff, and an adequate referral base.

Resources Not Utilized

All resources—including staff, equipment, finances, and so on—must be examined. Are staff members being employed to their fullest potential? Does the agency need to expand the use of computers in the office to do more data analysis? Could the agency sell some of the manuals, teaching tools, and forms that have been developed?

Standards

Standards are guidelines by which an agency or staff member should function. With the stronger movement toward accreditation of home health agencies by the National League for Nursing and the Joint

Commission on Accreditation of Hospitals, standards will be used more. Agencies already are reviewed according to standards for Medicare certification. Associations such as the National Association of Home Care publish standards by which an agency should function. There are also professional standards of practice for staff. The American Nurses' Association has published *Home Health Standards* to guide the practice of registered nurses in home care.

Agencies must use standards to conduct an in-house review before outside reviews are done. Examiners will identify problem areas that the agency must address.

Values of the Client

Planning and problem identification are based on distinct values of the organization and client. Values are conceptions of what is desirable or worthy and are utilized as criteria for choice or preference (Blum, 1974). Values include the religious, social, political, and ethnic beliefs of individuals. Values influence a client's usage of an agency and what services clients request. The values of staff members also influence how services or duties are carried out.

Unmet Needs

The audit is helpful in identifying unmet needs. From analyzing the components of the audit, the agency can identify areas where clients need a particular service and no one in the community is meeting that need. For example, the increase in mothers who work outside the home has created the need for someone to care for sick children versus since the present system of day care does not allow sick children to come to day care centers.

Conditions

Not all problems can be solved by one agency or group. Once problems or opportunities have been identified, the question must be asked: Is this something our agency can do something about? For example the agency can do something about inadequate staff and expanding services. It is more difficult to address the total reimbursement system under Medicare. Often problems need to be referred to other groups.

Inadequate housing is often seen by health staff in the home. This is an area where referral to the Department of Housing and Urban Development or a housing authority would be most beneficial in assisting the client. The agency can only deal with the problem of continuing to give quality care in poor housing, since quality care is something the agency can control.

Priorities

Priorities of the agency need to be considered when analyzing problems. From the problems that have been identified, priority may be assigned by the following steps (Blum, 1974):

1. Indicate which items are to be implemented first.
2. Indicate which items are then to receive no further consideration.
3. Indicate which item is to receive the major share of resources.
4. Indicate whether the activities called for by the high-priority items can be accomplished.
5. Indicate which among the high-ranking items are to get the go-ahead, the timetable for implementation, and the proportion of resources to be used.

GOALS AND OBJECTIVES

The next step is to identify goals and objectives. Goals and objectives reflect and operationalize the institutional strategy (Thieme et al., 1981). Goals are broad, general statements of the aim, purpose, or intent to be achieved. Some examples of goals are (1) to increase the number of referrals for skilled nursing care from XYZ hospital, (2) to improve the availability of physical therapists to the agency, and (3) to decrease the number of denials for reimbursement.

The goal states the broad purpose but does not give specifics as to how the goal will be obtained. That is the purpose of the objectives. Objectives specify and operationalize the strategy. Objectives state (1) who will experience (2) what change or benefit, (3) how much, and (4) how soon (Green et al., 1988). Other criteria for objectives are that they should be written, measurable, results oriented, realistic, specific, acceptable to all, flexible, consistent with each other, and challenging. Examples of an objective for goal number 1 above are

1. The number of referrals for skilled nursing care from XYZ hospital will increase over last year's figure according to the following schedule:

    a. By 20% the first year

    b. By 40% the second year

2. The proportion of home health care users that are satisfied with (a) the quality of care (b) scheduling and (c) the cooperation of staff will be raised to at least 90% in the next year.

These objectives state very specifically what action will be taken. From the objectives, specific strategies must be developed to determine how to reach the goals and objectives previously defined by the agency.

STRATEGY DEVELOPMENT

Strategies range from the very simple to the complex. Simple strategy development requires common sense planning. Highly sophisticated strategy development tests statistically whether an idea is feasible. Strategies, whether simple or complex, indicate where the major efforts of the organization should be directed in order to attain stated objectives.

At any given time, a substantial number of strategy alternatives are available. In exploring strategies, one technique for starting the process is to brainstorm. This method allows the planners to state any solution regardless of the reality of being able to carry it out. All the ideas are put out on the table and then evaluated as to which look most feasible. Often different ideas can be merged, or one idea spawns another. When evaluating the reality or feasibility of a strategy, there are six criteria that should be applied: time, power, finances, resources, information, and interest.

The aspect of time is evaluated to determine whether the strategy can be accomplished within the given time frame. In terms of power, the agency examines whether the strategy has the support of powerful people or whether the agency has enough power to enforce it. Finances concern the financial resources needed and the availability of funds. Resources pertain to the staff, time, skill, equipment, and knowledge needed. Are these elements present in the agency already, or must these resources be added? Information includes the availability of all the data necessary to make an informed decision. For example, if the agency wants to target the elderly in the community, are there sources of information that identify who and where the elderly are in the community? Determining how interested someone or the administration is in the strategy presented is important. If there is no interest on the part of the individuals who would carry out the project or those who authorize the project, there will be lack of cooperation.

From the loosely structured brainstorming strategy, we go to the rational approach to strategic planning. This method uses a continuum of strategic program options (Crompton and Lamb, 1986). The continuum ranges from developing new programs to terminating existing programs. Table 6.3 illustrates this continuum.

For each area on the continuum, there are different marketing strategies that could be used. For new programs, new markets must be reached through modifying current programs or diversifying into new markets. For modifying existing programs, the agency needs to use strategies that will improve the program for the existing customer. The agency can also try to reach new markets through modification of their programs or services.

Existing programs should be tailored to getting greater client support in a particular market. The emphasis should be on improving the efficiency of a program and on targeting new markets for the services.

Reduction strategies concern reducing resources for an existing product or service. This may mean reducing staff, shortening hours of service, or reducing the different types of services.

The last strategy is to terminate the existing service or program. This is a painful strategy for most agencies. Often there is a lot of opposition to this type of solution. It must be remembered, though,

Table 6.3   Strategic Program Continuum

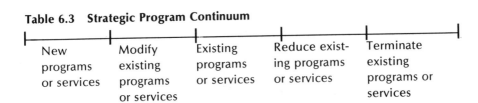

that to keep up in the marketplace old services often have to be eliminated so that new services can be implemented. It is better to terminate some programs or services than to stretch staff too thin.

One other method of strategy planning is called portfolio analysis. Like an investor's portfolio of stocks and bonds, an agency's portfolio of programs usually includes some that should be given additional support, some that should be maintained at their present level of support, some that should be modified, and some that should be terminated (Crompton and Lamb, 1986).

The paralysis of a portfolio employs a matrix. The two dimensions examined are demand for the service and market share. Figure 6.1 illustrates how this matrix can be used in home care.

In this matrix, skilled care for which there is a high demand and for which the agency has a high market share should be promoted vigorously. Homemaker services is an area that the agency should expand into. If this agency does not expand into homemaker services, another agency will do so to meet the high demand. Occupational therapy has no large demand, but the agency has a large part of the market. Resources should be allocated simply to maintain the service. In the area of hospice, there is low opportunity for growth, and the agency has a low share of the market. The service is one that could be terminated to allow the services that have a high market share and a high demand to expand.

These different types of strategy development can be used by an agency to meet its goals and objectives. The important point is not which model is used but that each strategy must be carefully evaluated to enable the agency to best use its resources. By examining the various strategies, the priority or most plausible strategy can be focused on and developed.

| | | Market Share | |
		High	Low
Demand for Service	High	Skilled care	Homemakers
	Low	Occupational therapy	Hospice

Figure 6.1. Portfolio matrix.

CONCLUSION

Problem identification is meaningless without action toward a solution. Such action is initiated through planning.

Planning can be done within a variety of frameworks. Various planning modes are laissez-fiare, disjointed incrementalism, allocative, problem solving, exploitive, explorative, normative, and the total planning. The type of model used depends on how the agency views planning. If the agency has a tendency to react to present conditions, laissez-faire or disjointed incrementalism would be the framework. In contrast, if an agency wants to plan for the future, they would use a problem-solving or exploitive mode.

Planning is done to identify what type of strategy the agency wants to select. There are four types: market penetration (obtaining a bigger share of the current market), market development (finding new targets), product development (changing or improving existing services), and diversification (finding new services). These strategies are kept in mind when the audit data is analyzed for opportunities or problems.

The analysis of the audit examines what has changed, discrepancies, weaknesses and strengths of the agency, resource utilization, standards, values and unmet needs of clients, and conditions the agency can do something about. The last step is to establish the agency's priorities. Various strategies are then developed and evaluated to address the problems. Each strategy must be carefully evaluated to enable the agency to best use its resources.

REFERENCES

Blum, H. *Planning for Health.* New York: Human Sciences Press, 1974.

Braden, C. *Community Health: A System and Approach*, New York: Appleton-Century-Crofts, 1976.

Cromptom, J., Lamb, C. *Marketing and Social Services.* New York: John Wiley & Sons, 1986.

Friedman, J. A conceptual model for the analysis of planning behavior *Administrative Science Quarterly.* 12(September 1967):225–252.

Green, L., Krueter, M., Deeds, S., Partridge, K. *Health Education Planning.* Palo Alto, CA: Mayfield, 1980.

Rubright, R., MacDonald, D. *Marketing Health and Human Services.* Rockville, MD: Aspen, 1981.

Thieme, C., Wilson, T., Long, D. Strategic planning for hospitals under regulation in *Strategic Planning in Health Care Management*. Flexner, W., Berkowitz E., M. Brown (eds.). Rockville, MD: Aspen, 1981, 13.

7

Implementation Phase

The conversion of plans into policy and practice is one of the main reasons for the market planning process. Activating programs calls for a sequence of steps to be performed and integrated into the agency's policies and practices.

One of the first steps in implementation requires gaining acceptance of the plan by both internal and external constituencies. Seeking to modify the perspectives of key publics or their representatives must be seen as a legitimate function of strategy planning (Crompton and Lamb, 1986).

Anytime ideas or plans are initiated there is a natural tendency for resistance to occur. VonOech (1986: 135) tells how an individual can carry an idea from the world of what if to the world of action. The greatest enemies of action are fear and lack of confidence. VanOech calls the idea implementation steps the "warrior's battle cry:"

Be bold
Put together your plan
Put a fire in your belly
Put a lion in your heart
Get going
Capitalize on your resources
Sharpen your sword
Know what you're selling
Strengthen your shield
Follow through
Use your energy wisely
Get up when you get knocked down
Savor your victories and learn from your defeats

If these steps are followed, acceptance of a plan has a high success rate.

One of the more concrete ways to reduce resistance to change is through participation of staff in the planning and implementation of the project. Zaltman and Duncan (1977: 92) elaborate on how participation and change interact:

1. Participation lessens feelings of alienation from those causing change.

2. Participation enhances staff feelings of control over decisions affecting them.

3. Communication among different groups within the target group is stimulated and facilitated.

4. Participants become more socialized into the thinking and operation of the group causing change.

STRATEGIES FOR IMPLEMENTATION

Strategies can be used to introduce change that occurs from the development of a new service, adjustment of an existing service, or discontinuation of a service. Burack and Torda (1979) suggest eight steps to use when implementing new ideas:

1. Communicate the idea to management that will implement the idea.
2. Develop technical and procedural plans.
3. Develop training methods for management.
4. Formulate a control system.
5. Communicate change to all personnel.
6. Prepare people for individual change.
7. Launch the program.
8. Redirect the idea.

Communicating to Managers

The first step is for the board of directors or administrator of the agency to communicate the idea to those managers or supervisors involved with implementing the idea. Too often plans are fully developed before supervisors or managers know about the proposed change. This group will also become the planning group that helps obtain input from the staff and deflect some of the resistance to the program or idea to be implemented. That is why it is essential for the managerial staff to know about ideas that are to be implemented.

Developing Plans

From this step technical and procedural plans are developed. For each implementation activity, the following questions must be answered in a detailed plan:

Who: individual responsible for the activity

What: task that needs to be done

Why: objectives stated

When: time frame of activity

Where: location of development and implementation

How: materials and resources needed

Answering these questions allows the development of an implementation strategy that can be scheduled on worksheets. The steps in developing an implementation strategy are detailed in Table 7.1.

Implementation worksheets can take many forms. The worksheet allows the marketer to be quite clear about the specific tasks, the time period required for completion, and what individual is going to be responsible. Flow charts, Gantt charts, and narratives are all styles of worksheets utilized and are discussed next.

Flow Charts

Flow charts are diagrams that show the steps needed to complete a certain project. It is harder in a flow diagram than a narrative to assign specific responsibility. Figure 7.1 illustrates a flow diagram of developing a health consulting firm. Time frames and responsibilities can be defined at the side of a diagram such as this. When developing flow charts, different symbols designate different activities. Figure 7.2

Table 7.1   Development of Implementation Strategy

1. Clearly specify assignments.
2. Assign someone responsibility for the whole project and coordination of staff
3. Identify all beginning steps before activity (e.g., write budget, put ad in paper).
4. List steps in the order they need done.
5. Check to be sure all steps are there.
6. Determine dates when activity should begin and end.
7. Check dates to allow enough time for activities.
8. Identify any potential problems.
9. Specify what resources will be needed and their source.
10. Make sure those involved know what is expected of them and by when.

Source: National Heart, Lung and Blood Institute. *Handbook for Improving High Blood Pressure Control in the Community.* Washington, DC: Government Printing Office, 1977, 36.

Figure 7.1. Health planning model (next page).

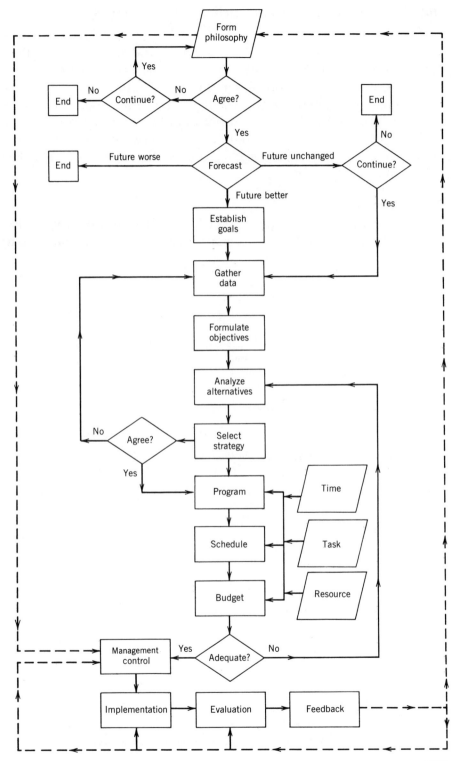

explains the different types of symbols found in Figure 7.1. Flow charting allows someone to quickly see the whole process step by step.

An example of such a process in the field of home health care is the development of a new service. The flow chart allows someone to see how the program will develop rather than to read a narration of the plan. Figure 7.3 shows how an objective to develop physical therapy services for a home health agency can be displayed using the flow chart method.

Gantt Charts

Gantt charts detail the activities of projects. An example of a Gantt chart is found in Table 7.2. This chart includes the tasks that need to

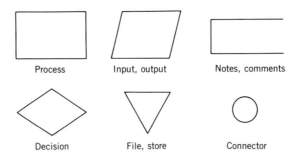

Figure 7.2. *Flow-charting symbols.*

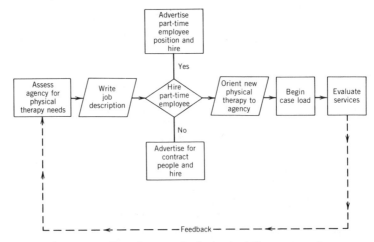

Figure 7.3. *Development of physical therapy services.*

be done, the resources needed, who is responsible, the due date, a check-off column indicating completion, and a comment column. Tasks of the project, such as "request permission from the board of directors to implement project A," are defined. The question then is asked: What resources do I need to accomplish that task? Items such as a secretary, figures from surveys, and the completed report are included. Whose responsibility to carry this function out is specified next. It is helpful to draw a line through the person's name or put a check by it to indicate that the person has been told it is his or her responsibility to complete the task. When many activities are going on in the agency, it is easy to forget whether someone has been told. This procedure prevents the arrival of the due date without the report. The due date is specified and should be realistic. You can always expect the unexpected to happen. Allow extra time. When the task is completed it can be checked off. It makes the planner feel good to look at a plan and see all those completed check marks. The last column is for any notes the planner wants to jot down.

Narrative

The narrative form resembles a "to do" list. The activities are listed, and dates are assigned for deadlines. Table 7.3 illustrates this type of format.

This form is the most basic of implementation strategies. It does include who is responsible for what task or what resources are needed. It is a good design to use if an agency has not committed its planning to paper before. It at least formalizes the steps and due dates for a project. This type of worksheet is helpful for a staff member to use when presenting a plan to a manager about the implementation of a new idea. This allows the manager to see all the steps needed and indicates that the staff member has actually thought through the whole process.

The method the agency chooses to use depends on its individual preference. The important thing is that the agency should write down the steps so the whole project can be visualized. The steps cannot be kept in someone's head but need to be shared with all who are involved.

Developing Training Methods

When new ideas are generated and resources are examined in planning, often new skills are needed. It is important to train

TABLE 7.2
IMPLEMENTATION WORKSHEET

Task	Resources	Due date	Done	Comments

Table 7.3   Narrative Worksheet

Tasks	Due Date
Activity: Create Homemaker Services	
Develop proposal for homemaker services	1/30
Request funds	2/15
Hire staff	3/1
Train and orient staff	3/25
Begin services	4/1

managers and supervisors how to handle change because staff members often pattern their behavior after that of supervisors. If staff members see that the nursing supervisor is resistant to adding more homemaker services, you can anticipate similar behavior from a large percentage of the staff.

People who have the respect of others should be sought out to pave the way for change. Giving these people additional training in listening skills, communicating ideas and feelings effectively, and handling conflict helps managers work better with their staff.

Formulating a Control System

Designing a control system is closely related to step two of the implementation phase, when plans and timetables are defined. When plans are developed, it is important to monitor how well they are being implemented and whether the program is on schedule. Too often staff members are not told whether a planned change will be a permanent or temporary situation. If they know when an idea is to be implemented and what will happen and if they have input as the program is implemented, resistance to change decreases. One of the most important aspects of this step is to make sure that feedback mechanisms are established as a system is implemented and at the completion of the program or service.

Communicating with Personnel

Communication is one of the most important aspects of implementation. All personnel should know that new services or ideas are going to be implemented in the agency. How management communicates the timetable for a change and what management says are very important in ensuring staff support. Personnel do not like to be told at a Monday staff meeting that new services are starting the next day.

Although information may be accurate and well intentioned, it sometimes fails to accomplish the desired results. Messages should not be given in numerous memos and communications. Rather, a single message should give all the information about the new idea, including what it means to the agency and the employee, the time frame for implementation, and the feedback mechanisms. This message should first be given to managers and supervisors so they can reinforce the idea when the administrator discusses it with employees. Rather than using a "trickle down" system, the administration should announce the changes to demonstrate administrative support for the idea and to show how important it is that the staff is kept informed.

Individual Change

Because new programs or ideas often affect staff, management should clearly determine what changes, if any, are expected of staff members and managers. Training programs should be initiated that will aid the staff in implementing new tasks. For example, if an agency has decided not to contract with intravenous therapy companies but to train its own nursing staff to do intravenous therapy, considerable training or refresher courses should be offered to prepare the nurses for their new role.

Also, letting staff members rehearse or practice their new roles or responsibilities before they are on their own is helpful. A buddy system works well to make the staff more comfortable. Positive reinforcement is important from all levels of employees to encourage people through the change process until they gain confidence in their new roles and responsibilities.

Launching the Program

An agency can never anticipate all aspects of launching a new program. The important thing is to get the program off and running and have the control system well in place to locate problems early in a new program.

Too often good ideas are planned but never implemented. If careful planning has been done, programs or ideas can be implemented and monitored. Programs can be modified: they are not engraved in stone.

It is important that the atmosphere in this phase is one in which people feel free to comment on how the program is going and on problems that are developing. Management needs to ask for feedback and encourage it.

Redirection

If an open communication system is established early in implementing a strategy, redirection is relatively easy. The system has gathered the needed feedback from staff, records, data gathered in the service, and management.

From all this information, decisions can be made as to any

alterations needed in the program. Feedback can also be obtained on how the planned alterations would solve the problem and on other possible solutions. Because of the rapid change in the health care delivery system, no program, service, or idea can remain unchanged. Agencies must have the ability to redirect services.

CONCLUSION

The conversion of plans into practice is one of the main reasons for the market planning process. Activating programs calls for a sequence of steps to be performed and integrated into the agency's policies and practices.

Anytime new plans or ideas are initiated, there is a natural tendency for resistance to occur. Ideas to overcome change include reducing fear and increasing the level of confidence of personnel. Other suggestions are to increase staff participation in planning and implementation.

A step-by-step approach to implementing ideas suggests that management needs to communicate with staff about new ideas, develop implementation plans, develop training methods for management, formulate a control system, communicate change to all personnel, and prepare people for individual change. The program then is launched, and redirection of the program is done if needed.

Flow charts, Gantt charts, and narratives are all tools to help in the development of a plan. By using these tools and steps, a marketer is able to implement new ideas and programs with the least resistance.

REFERENCES

Burack, E., Torda, F. *The Manager's Guide to Change.* Belmont, CA: Lifetime Learning Publications, 1979.

Crompton, J., Lamb, C. *Marketing Government and Social Services.* New York: John Wiley & Sons, 1986.

Fox, D., Fox, R. Strategic planning for nursing, *Journal of Nursing Administration.* (May 1983):11–17. Vol. 13, No. 5

National Heart, Lung and Blood Institute. *Handbook for Improving High Blood Pressure Control in the Community.* Washington, DC: Government Printing Office, 1977.

VonOech, R. *A Kick in the Seat of the Pants.* New York: Perennial Library, 1986, 135.

Williams, S., Developing a nursing consulting firm. Unpublished paper presented to the American Public Health Association, Dallas, November 16, 1983.

Zaltman, G., Duncan, R. *Strategies for Planned Change.* New York: John Wiley & Sons, 1977:92.

8

Control
Phase

Evaluation is the process of determining the value or amount of success in achieving a predetermined objective (American Public Health Association, 1960). Evaluation is not a set of arbitrary applications. Rather, it is a rerun of the planning process after the results are in hand to learn whether one got what was intended, at the price, in the amounts, and in the way specified and whether it is still wanted (Warren, 1973).

PURPOSES AND TYPES OF EVALUATION

Suchman (1967: 141) enumerates the specific purposes of evaluation:

1. Evaluation measures the effectiveness of a program.
2. Evaluation examines the efficiency of the program.
3. Evaluation, properly used and designed, is a quality-control device.
4. Evaluation identifies side effects.
5. Evaluation helps to identify the strengths and weaknesses in the processes used to carry out the program so that they can either be corrected or built into strengths.
6. Evaluation permits testing the effectiveness of the organizational structure and/or modes of operation.
7. Evaluation develops a critical attitude within the program.
8. Evaluation is a means of providing explicit accountability to the public.

Knutson (1969: 42) looks at evaluation from the point of view of the organization and states that program evaluation may be undertaken to

1. Demonstrate to others that the program is worthwhile
2. Determine whether or not a program is moving in the right direction
3. Determine whether the needs for which the program is designed are being satisfied
4. Justify past or projected expenditures
5. Determine the costs of a program in terms of money or human effort

6. Obtain evidence that may be helpful in demonstrating to others what is already believed to be true regarding the effectiveness of a program

7. Gain support for program expansion

8. Compare different types of programs in terms of their relative effect

9. Compare different program methods or approaches in terms of effect

10. Satisfy someone who has demanded evidence of effect

There are two levels of evaluation: formative and summative. Each can address the issues described above. Formative evaluation requires collecting and sharing information while the program is being installed. The formative evaluator works to provide the program planners and staff with information to help adjust the program to the setting and improve it. In contrast, the summative evaluator examines the total impact of a program either at the conclusion of a developmental period or when the program has been in operation for awhile (Morris and Fitz-Gibbon, 1978).

Formative evaluation requires monitoring of a system as it is being implemented. The evaluator collects information about what the program is achieving and how it is perceived by clients and staff. There is not always a formal method of collecting such data. Much of this evaluation is done through observation, selected interviews, and documents already gathered. The purpose of this type evaluation is to find problems early and resolve them before a program has been in place for a long period of time.

The more formal method of evaluation is the summative evaluation. This method examines the program or project after it has been implemented and evaluates how well the original predetermined objective was met. The evaluator examines whether there has been an increase of awareness or an increase in the number of referrals from XYZ Hospital. Blum (1974) describes five steps in this process:

1. Clarify goal and objectives.

2. Select or design measurement instruments or other procedures to collect data.

3. Collect data.

4. Summarize and analyze data.

5. Interpret data and conclude what it shows.

DATA COLLECTION METHODS

Once the original predetermined goals and objectives are examined and clarified if necessary, the evaluator is ready to consider how to measure those objectives. There are many different data collection methods, including polls, surveys, questionnaires, observation, focus groups, financial records, health records, and unsolicited comments.

Table 8.1 illustrates various survey methods and criteria to use when trying to choose what type of method to use. When using questionnaires, surveys, and polls, the evaluator must decide on the format of questioning and what type of questions to ask. Open-ended questions are very general, for example, What service from our agency are you most satisfied with? Closed-ended questions ask, for example, What service from our agency are you most satisfied with: skilled nursing, physical therapy, homemaker services, or none of the above? Table 8.2 identifies strengths and weaknesses of open-ended and close-ended questions and when to use each.

Another data collection method is observation. Observation can be a helpful tool to see how staff members are using a new treatment procedure in the home or how they interact with a client in the home. Even if observation is done, there should be defined questions that the observation is measuring.

Table 8.1   Characteristics/General Evaluation Criteria of Survey Methods

Characteristics and Criteria	Mailed Questionnaire	Telephone Survey	Personal Interview	Focus Group
Expense	Low	Low to medium	High	Medium
Response rate	Low	Medium to high	High	High
Completion time	Medium	Low (shortest)	High (longest)	Low to medium
Versatility	Low	Medium	High	High
Amount of information	Medium	Low	High	Medium
Clarity for respondent	Low	Medium	High	High

Source: Cooper, P., Hisrich, R. Marketing research for health services: understanding and applying various techniques. *Journal of Health Care Marketing.* 7(1987):54–61. Published by the American Marketing Association.

Table 8.2 Construction of Open-Ended and Closed-Ended Questions

Strengths	Weaknesses	When to Use
Open-Ended Questions		
Wide range of responses	Hard to get responses of limited length	To expand an idea
Response not influenced by category	Difficult to record	Cannot list all responses
One question can lead to another	Chance of investigator bias	To search for feelings, beliefs, and attitudes
Build on where the person is going	Time consuming	More detail or depth needed
Much easier to construct	Expensive to code and tabulate	Evaluator does not want to bias by category
More specific questions	Great coding variability	Information needed beyond recall
Makes people feel important	Difficult to generalize hypothesis	Time is available
		As an ice breaker
		To get unaided knowledge
		To add "anything else"
Closed-Ended Questions		
Much easier to use	Very time consuming to develop	For large population
Gives respondent structure	Results can be skewed	Time is a factor
Less variability of responses	Answers box people in	Data need statistical analysis
Easier to compare	Make sure all answers are plausible	Bias of open-ended questions could alter responses
Data easier to tabulate	Does not allow for expression of additional information	Easier to compare
More applicable to statistical analysis	Hard to have choices clearly stated with no research bias	Easier to categorize people
More approaches can be used	Ordering of questions important	You have control of responses
		Avoid subjective evaluation
		Get more information
		Ease in structuring respondents

Focus groups are a technique that grew out of the group therapy method of psychiatrists. The concept is based on the assumption that people who share a problem will be more willing to talk about it amid the security of others sharing the problem. The procedure brings together people in a discussion group atmosphere to discuss feelings, attitudes, and perceptions about the topic being discussed (Bellinger et al., 1976).

Other data collection resources are financial and health records. These data are especially helpful when examining the cost as well as the usage of a program.

Financial records can help to identify costs of the program as well as any unexpected expenses. Cost per visits, cost of personnel, administrative costs, and marketing costs are all examples of financial data that can be used to help evaluate.

Using health records for evaluation adds utilization data. From records, the type of health conditions seen most frequently and the procedures required can be determined. Records also give the source of referral and type of payment. Social data are also available. These data are helpful in examining who refers and who should be target markets. Profiling the client that receives the services is another use of social data. All of these data help the agency to evaluate services, usage, and types of skills needed.

The last data collection tool consists of unsolicited comments. To use such information, there must be a mechanism by which clients are able to comment on their level of satisfaction. This mechanism can be a postcard or a suggestion to clients that they are free to comment at any time to a person in the agency who has been designated the client contact person. Letting the client know the agency wants to hear comments will facilitate this process.

CRITERIA FOR EVALUATION

Combined with the various data that are collected is the need for determining what should be evaluated. Blum (1974) and Arnold (1971) define six evaluation questions that need to be answered to do a summative evaluation. The process begins with the stated objective. Then six questions are answered:

1. Activity: Is the operation working?
2. Criteria: Is it operating according to a prescribed manner or criteria?

3. Efficiency: Is the operation working at the cost agreed upon?

4. Effectiveness: How well is the program producing the desired outputs?

5. Outcome validity: How well has the intervention achieved the consequences or purposes for which the outputs were designed?

6. Desirability: Does the desired result actually serve the overall best interest of the encompassing system?

The steps in evaluation examine a range of factors. All steps should be examined, whether briefly or formally, to accomplish the best evaluation of the marketing effort.

Step 1: Activity

The first step in the evaluation process determines whether the program exists and what activity is going on. The Gantt chart or other schedule used for program implementation, described in Chapter 7, provides a guide to see if all tasks have been accomplished. Table 8.3 shows an example of how program implementation charts are used for evaluation. The column marked "done" is analyzed to determine whether the activity is being done and the causes of delay, if any. This example shows that the agency currently is in the evaluation phase but all other activities have been accomplished.

Step 2: Criteria

It must be determined not only whether the system is working, but whether it operates in the prescribed manner or according to criteria or standards. Standards that affect home health care are accreditation and certification standards. Payment can be denied an agency when criteria are not met in delivering care. Application of the standards often leads to a consideration of accessibility of the program to the target population, control over costs, and other criteria that measure the delivery of services.

Step 3: Efficiency

Efficiency is a measure of the degree to which the agency produces the output as inexpensively as it could (Crompton and Lamb, 1986). The common measurement in health care is often providing a service and counting the number of clients who have utilized the service. It is also

Table 8.3 Implementation Worksheet

Task	Resources	Responsibility	Due	Done	Evaluation
Develop proposal for homemaker services	Staff coordinator of home services, finance director, marketing director	Coordinator of home services	1/7/88	1/30/88	Delayed due to new regulations
Request funds	Board of directors, administrator, finance director	Administrator	3/1/88	4/1/88	Board approved minus $2,000, budget adjusted
Hire staff	Personnel director, coordinator of home services, newspapers, radio	Personnel, coordinator of home services	4/1/88	5/15/88	Is problem; enough applicants
Train and orient staff	Staff, consultant, coordinator of home services, manual from the National Association of Home Care	Coordinator of home services	4/15/88	6/1/88	Used prepared manual, good; need more local examples
Begin services	Homemakers, coordinator of home services	All	4/18/88	6/5/88	Services requested
Market services	Marketing director, coordinator of home services, all staff	Marketing director	4/15/88	6/1/88	Good flow of clients; stress paying clients, some nonpaying
Evaluate after 2 months	Coordinator of home services, finance director, marketing director	Coordinator of home services	6/15/88		

helpful to consider the proportion or number of clients satisfied with the service per dollar or per employee dollar. Whenever efficiency measures concentrate on any dimension of service, such as hospice care, personnel interpret this as a signal of management's priority and concentrate on the activities measured. Also, efficiency can become excessive when agencies cannot function according to the standards they have set because of cost effectiveness.

Step 4: Effectiveness

The measurement of effectiveness involves finding out if relevant segments of the public are satisfied with the benefits the program offers. This step examines the impact of the program with such questions as (1) To what extent—and why—are program recipients better off, worse off, or unchanged as a result of the program activity?, (2) Can the results of the program be explained by some alternative process that does not include the program?, and (3) Is the program having some effects that were not intended (Rossi et al., 1979)?

It is also important in this step to measure clients' satisfaction and benefits they have received from the services. Table 8.4 presents samples of various ways questions are asked of clients.

Step 5: Outcome Validity

To measure outcome validity, the agency explores how well it has achieved the purposes for which the outputs were identified. The evaluator examines the original objectives to see if the programs carried out have accomplished them. For example, if one objective was to increase the number of referrals, the evaluator examines whether the strategies implemented have resulted in an increase.

Step 6: Desirability

The final step in evaluation examines whether the program serves the best interests of the system. The program that was implemented needs to be examined to see how well it fits with other programs of the agency, community, and society. With the competitiveness of today's marketplace, the agency may know it has a good program that will benefit society but ten other agencies may also be providing the same service. Consideration must be given to whether the program should

Table 8.4 Sample Survey Questions

Sample 1 Client Survey

1. Did your nurse tell you about the treatment that you will need at home?
   ____ Yes   ____ No
2. What did you like most about XYZ Agency?

Sample 2: Physician Questionnaire

1. On what basis do you decide which agency to refer clients to:
   ____ Client request or preference
   ____ Specialty services
   ____ Agency reputation
   ____ Type of services available
   ____ Cost
   ____ Hours of coverage
   ____ Other
2. What services do patients currently need that are not available?

Sample 3: Client Questionnaire

1. How would you rate the attitude of agency personnel involved with your care.
   ( ) Good   ( ) Fair   ( ) Poor
2. Did agency personnel spend their time in the most efficient manner?
   ____ Yes   ____ No
   Comments:

Sample 4: Client Scale

1. The nurse explains things in simple language.

1	2	3	4	5
Strongly disagree	Disagree	Neutral	Agree	Strongly agree

2. The nurse is understanding in listening to client's problem.

1	2	3	4	5
Strongly disagree	Disagree	Neutral	Agree	Strongly agree

Sample 5: Service Evaluation

1. In general, how satisfied were the members of your family with the care they received from hospice?

1	2	3	4	5
Very dissatisfied	Somewhat dissatisfied	Somewhat satisfied	Very satisfied	Not appropriate

2. In general, how satisfied were the members of your family with your nurse's availability?

1	2	3	4	5
Very dissatisfied	Somewhat dissatisfied	Somewhat satisfied	Very satisfied	Not appropriate

continue or whether money should be given to another project in which fewer agencies are involved.

MODIFICATION

Any form of evaluation leads the agency to consider what modifications should be made in a program. Areas of weakness are identified from the evaluation, and the agency then determines what specific modifications are needed. Modifications can be made in the areas of: objectives, goals, personnel, leadership, methods of delivery, cost, resources, training, or evaluation methods. It is important to remember that market planning is not a fixed activity. Rather, it is a cycle that continually moves the agency forward into the future (see Figure 8.1).

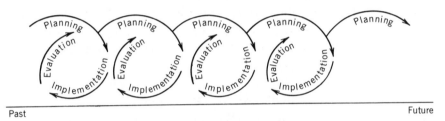

Past   Future

Figure 8.1. The marketing cycle.

CONCLUSION

Evaluation is not an arbitrary process but one of carefully planned steps to determine whether if the agency has achieved a predetermined objective. Evaluation measures the effectiveness of a program, identifies its strengths and weaknesses, and provides for accountability to the public.

Two types of evaluation can be done: formative and summative. Formative evaluation examines the program as it is being implemented. Its focus is on adjusting the program and improving it while it is being implemented. Summative evaluation examines the program after it has been implemented to determine how well the original predetermined objectives were met.

Data collection for evaluation involves the use of a variety of methods, including polls, surveys, questionnaires, observation, focus groups, financial records, health records, and unsolicited comments. Using the data gathered by these means, the agency determines what it wants to evaluate. The six areas of summative evaluation are activity, criteria, efficiency, effectiveness, outcome validity, and desirability.

Once the agency performs the evaluation, modifications often have to be made. This is the purpose of evaluation: to find out how to make the program better. Modifications start the planning process and help move the agency toward meeting the next opportunity.

REFERENCES

American Nurses' Association. *Home Health Care Standards.* Kansas City, Missouri, 1987.

American Public Health Association. Glossary of administrative terms in public health. *American Journal of Public Health.* 50(1960):225–226.

Arnold, M. Evaluation: a parallel process to planning in *Administering Health Systems: Issues and Perspectives.* Blakenship, A. M., Hess, J. (eds.). New York: Aldine Atherton, 1971.

Bellinger, D., Bernhardt, K., Goldstucker, J. *Qualitative Research in Marketing.* Chicago: American Marketing Association, 1976, 7–28.

Blum, H. *Planning for Health: Development and Application of Social Change Theory.* New York: Human Sciences Press, 1974.

Cooper, P., Hirsich, R. Marketing research for health services: understanding and applying various techniques. *Journal of Health Care Marketing.* 7(1987): 54–61.

Crompton, J., Lamb, C. *Marketing Government and Social Services.* New York: John Wiley & Sons, 1986.

Knutson, A. Evaluation for what? in *Program Evaluation in the Health Field.* Schulberg, H. (ed.). New York: Human Sciences Press, 1969, 42.

Morris, L., Fitz-Gibbon, C. *Evaluator's Handbook.* Beverly Hills, CA: Sage Publications, 1978.

Rossi, P., Freeman, H., Wright, S. *Evaluation: A systematic Approach.* Beverly Hills, CA: Sage Publications, 1979, 33.

Suchman, E. *Evaluative Research.* New York: Russel Sage Foundation, 1967, 141.

Warren, R. *Truth, Love and Social Change.* Chicago: Rand McNally, 1973.

PART 3

Marketing Your Agency Effectively: Tools and Personnel

9

Promotion

Promotion is communication that tells potential users about an agency's services and attempts to persuade them that the benefits the agency provides will satisfy their needs (Rubright and MacDonald, 1981). In marketing, promotional tools carry direct messages to targets. These messages reflect market objectives and strategies, and the tools are selected from an array of choices and funneled through four promotional channels: advertising, personal selling, public relations, and incentives.

Promotion is done through these channels and has four main purposes:

1. Inform: give clients basic information to make a decision; information includes name of the agency, location, telephone number, hours of the agency, and services offered.

2. Educate: inform public about what home care is and how it can use the services; goal is to get clients to value and thus want the services.

3. Persuade: clients not only need information but may need to be persuaded to use the services; persuaders are items such as quality of services, convenience of services, pleasantness of staff, and personal satisfaction with services.

4. Remind: since clients have alternatives to home care, the agency must remind clients and families that use of home care is a wise use of their resources.

COMMUNICATION PROCESS

Before the various channels of communication can be addressed, the communication process must be examined. Assael (1984: 203) stated that "any type of communication requires a source, a message, a means of transmitting the message, and a receiver." Figure 9.1 shows the elements involved in all communication. These elements are defined as follows:

Source: whoever wants to send a message

Encoding: putting thoughts into a form

Message: stating the benefits of the product or service and the objectives of the message

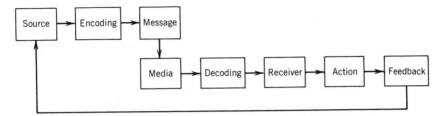

Figure 9.1. *Communication model.*

Media: communication channels through which the message is
  sent

Decoding: translation of the message for meaning by the receiver

Receiver: party that receives the message

Action: reaction of the receiver once he or she has been exposed to
  the message

Feedback: communication from the receiver, by his or her action,
  back to the sender

The agency has information it wants to share with a potential client group. The information that should be included begins the encoding process. The message is then built by stating the benefits of the services and the objective of the message. This message is distributed through various media. The potential client takes the message, translates it (decodes it for its meaning), and then determines what action to take. The action the agency wants is use of its services. Feedback is provided to the source by whatever action the client takes.

For communication to be successful, three conditions must be present. First, the message must be designed and delivered to gain the attention of the intended target audience. Second, the message must address the wants of the intended target audience and suggest a means of satisfying one or more of those wants. Third, the message must be appropriately positioned, which means that it must be related to and consistent with the existing knowledge and experience of a target market (Crompton and Lamb, 1986). Message development is further discussed later in this chapter.

For the communication process to work, it must use various channels to take the message to the public. Figure 9.2 diagrams the four channels of promotional communication: advertising, personal selling, public relations, and incentives.

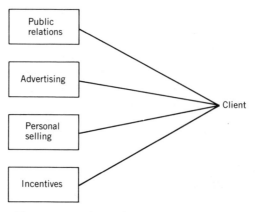

Figure 9-2. Channels of communication.

CHANNELS

Advertising

Advertising consists of nonpersonal forms of communication conducted through paid media under clear sponsorship (Kotler, 1982). Advertising is done to promote the agency's name, promote a service or product, and disseminate information about a particular service or event. It is sponsored by the agency to a target audience through varied media, such as television, radio, newspapers, magazines, direct mailings, circulars, novelties, and outdoor displays.

Public service announcements are a unique form of advertising that is not paid for by the agency. The air time or print space is donated by a radio or television network, a local station, or a newspaper. The agency does not have control over when the announcement will appear because the time is donated. The National Association of Home Care has produced several public service announcements on home care that can be purchased and used by a local agency. Some state associations of home care have produced public service announcement tapes that discuss home care issues in the particular state and can be purchased by agencies to use with their local stations. One such announcement used as its theme, "It's nice to be home. Health care is back home where it belongs."

Personal Selling

Personal selling is direct personal communication between a representative from the agency and a prospective client for the purpose of getting the client to use the agency's services. This method of communicating is increasingly used by home health agencies. It is important to remember that every time personnel interact in a professional capacity with present or prospective clientele, they are directly or indirectly communicating something about the agency and/or its services. This subject is explored further in Chapter 11.

Public Relations

Public relations is any unpaid form of news, editorial comment, or contact with people about an agency that is transmitted through mass media at no charge to the agency (Crompton and Lamb, 1986). This area is often confused with marketing. Kotler (1982: 381) differentiates public relations and marketing as follows:

1. Public relations is primarily a communication tool, whereas marketing also includes need assessment, product development, pricing, and distribution.
2. Public relations seeks to influence attitudes, whereas marketing tries to elicit specific behaviors such as purchasing, joining, and so on.
3. Public relations does not define the goals of the organization, whereas marketing is intimately involved in defining the business' mission, customers, and services.

Public relations people are the caretakers and enhancers of the agency's image. Commom examples of public relations are print or broadcast editorials and feature stories, health fairs, publications, radio talk shows, speeches, and telephone information services. The Visiting Nurses Association (VNA) of St. Louis currently has a telephone number called VNA-CARE that the public can call and ask a registered nurse questions on health matters.

Incentives

Incentives are something of financial or symbolic value that is added to an offer to encourage some behavioral response (Kotler, 1982). This type of promotion asks clients to take a course of action within a certain time frame. Methods used are coupons, contests, toll-free numbers, treasure hunts, specific communication responses (e.g., to mention an ad when they call), and discounts.

An example of this in the field of home care is a direct mail coupon that gives 10% off the first time someone uses homemaker services. One agency uses an educational brochure on how to select a home agency as an incentive for the general public to request, and then it also sends the potential client information about the agency.

MESSAGE DESIGN

As mentioned previously, for communication to be successful the message must be carefully constructed. In designing messages, the aim is to tailor the communication to a target situation in such a way as to be optimally effective and efficient (MacStravic, 1986). For every channel used there is a process of message development that is basic to all forms of communication. The message is developed with the old theme of who, what, where, when, how, and why in mind.

The "who" refers to both the target and the source of the message. The question that has to be examined is, Who is to be informed? Often the target audiences for promotional material are segments of the population. These targets could be older residents, working mothers, American Association of Retired Persons (AARP) members, or others. The second question involves identifying the source of the message. The source can be your agency or a spokesperson. The appearance of a well-known person as the source of the message may serve to attract a larger audience or a certain market segment. However, this method can also create problems of credibility. It is important that the spokesperson has a clear understanding of the service or agency so that he or she can give informed answers to questions.

The "what" of the message is specifying objectives of the message. The objective addresses a certain behavior, mind set, attitude, or knowledge that is to be achieved. Most objectives are informational: they serve to increase awareness, knowledge, or beliefs. Precisely stating the objective makes the message clearer.

The "where" of the message is where the audience will be when exposed to the message. The agency must be able to determine where the people will be, how they can be reached, and when they would be most receptive. For example, an ad on a 12:00 P.M. news report would probably not reach many elderly people living at home.

The timing of messages is the "when." Considerations for timing include the time of the year or month, how many times and how frequently to present a message, when a client is most receptive, and the rate of speed at which the message is communicated. All these factors must be examined in detail in considering the time factor.

The choice of media is the "how" of the message. There are many media choices from television to flyers to direct mailing to personal selling. Media choices are discussed in more detail later in this chapter.

The last area is the message content, or the "why." The "why" question addresses how the message should be worded to bring about the intended result.

Chapman (1985) feels that messages have maximum impact when they represent the value that the agency provides and that consumers are seeking. "Someone still makes house calls" is an example of a value-oriented home care slogan. It promotes the agency and imparts positive values that the client will want and respond to. In this phrase, the agency communicates its caring attitude and the unique character of its service.

The values of clients have great impact on the message and its content. If the message is written to address what is of value to the client, there is a high probability that the message will be successful.

Five Parts of a Message

A message has five parts: grabber, theme, body, hook and signature (MacStravic, 1986). Not all messages must have all five parts, but it is a good idea to think through all five. Each of the five parts is briefly described below:

Grabber: headline that grabs the attention of the intended audience

Theme: piece of information, feeling, or conclusion that the audience is expected to receive

Body: contains the theme and evidence, arguments, discussions, or descriptions that reinforce the theme

Hook: behavioral response requested as justified by the theme and body

Signature: sponsor's identification, logo, and/or slogan

Grabber

The grabber is considered one of the most important parts of the message. It is the headline that grabs the attention of the audience. If that attention is not obtained, the message is lost. A headline is typically short. The grabber tries to arouse curiosity or to single out a specific audience. "Wish to stop smoking?" singles out an audience that is interested in stopping smoking. Some grabbers, such as, "Are you ready for a change?" are designed to arouse curiosity. This causes the person to be curious about what is inside.

In writing a grabber, it is important to remember the values of clients. If a grabber says, "I love the VNA," it is selling this agency; if it says, "The VNA loves you," it conveys the message that care is delivered with a caring attitude (Chapman, 1985). Too often, health care agencies put their building or name on the front of promotional material. This does not convey any immediate value to the client. The examples below are grabber statements that will get the attention of the client since they reflect a value the client understands:

1. "Are you an unemployed nurse who would rather be working?" (radio message).
2. "Public health nurses are here to help you" (brochure).
3. "When it comes to health care, there's no place like home" (home care agency).
4. "How to keep your home safe for you and your family" (brochure on home safety).
5. "Children are special people and deserving of special care" (pediatric home care program).
6. "Professional rewards, personal freedom" (staff recruiting brochure for home care).
7. "Independence and home intravenous therapy: now you can have them both" (home care intravenous program).
8. "Expect the most from the best" (home care agency).

Theme

The theme builds on the grabber statement and conveys pieces of information, feelings, or conclusions that the audience is intended to draw. The information includes themes such as comprehensive care, skilled nursing, competent staff, and 24-hour availability and all the basic facts about the agency's services. Feelings and conclusions focus on how the agency wants someone to feel after they have read the promotional material. For example, the material may be designed to elicit the conclusion that home care is a practical solution and that it offers the family a helping hand, or it may generate a feeling of confidence that the family's loved one will get good care.

The creation of the marketing message should begin with the theme. The theme describes the desired effect; everything else is intended to create that effect. Often the theme is repeated in the same words in successive messages that are developed.

It is important to pretest a message to determine how people summarize what they have seen and heard. The intended theme can be evaluated based on what people remember and believe and what their overall feelings are about the message and the agency. If the theme the agency wants to communicate to the audience does not get across, it needs to be modified (MacStravic, 1986).

Body
The body of the message is the content between the grabber and the hook. It contains the theme but also supplies evidence, discussions, or descriptions that reinforce the theme. In the body, the agency details its comprehensive services, explains what 24-hour-a-day services mean, gives testimony from former patients about services, or presents an endorsement of the agency from someone else.

There is no absolute rule on the length of the body. For most messages, though, a short body keeps the interest of the reader. The length depends on the target audience.

The body, then, builds on the grabber and emphasizes the theme with evidence, explanation, or repetition of information. Finally, the body leads up to and prepares the way for the hook.

Hook
The purpose of promotion is to get the client to take some action. The hook is the response requested of the client. It is usually a request to call or write the agency or to try its services. Examples of hooks are

1. Call now.
2. Call VNA-CARE.
3. For your free information packet, call _____ .
4. Present this coupon and get a free _____ .
5. Ask a neighbor who's been there.
6. Please send me your free general information brochure on home health care.

Signature

The signature is the sponsor's identification, logo, and/or slogan. This is the final component of a message. The signature is intended to unite all the messages put out by an agency.

One very successful campaign has been that for Kleenex. As a result of this campaign, say, "Give me a Kleenex," not "Give me a facial tissue." The signature is reinforced everytime someone reaches for a Kleenex. Examples of slogans used in home health are "Care at a price you can afford," "Assisting each person to remain independent," "Caring for your children and family is important to you . . . it's important to us also," "Expect the best," "The one name for your home care needs," and "Personalized home care." It is important to place the slogan, logo, and identifying data on all materials that come from the agency. These items include letterhead, forms, brochures, ads, and novelty items. All of this reinforces to the client recognition of your agency's services.

MARKETING MESSAGES

MacLachlan (1983/1984: 51) summarizes this discussion of development of messages by giving suggestions for making marketing messages memorable and persuasive:

1. Use high-imagery words and pictures.
2. After the grabber, suggest a benefit gained or a problem avoided.
3. Use questions to arouse people's curiosity and to generate involvement.
4. Use familiar terms.
5. Provide an organizing sequence that will hold the message together.
6. Use specific rather than general terms.
7. Repeat key words and ideas that are central to the theme of the message.
8. Put the most important thoughts and words at the beginning.
9. Use concrete rather than abstract words and pictures rather than words.

10. Aim at one member of the family or group.

11. Tell the audience the implications of reaching the conclusion.

Now that channels of communication and message development have been discussed, the use of media to reach the public will be examined.

TOOLS

What promotional tools do you need? Is a brochure enough? Should you use novelty items? These are all questions the administrator of an agency often asks. Whatever tool is used, there are certain characteristics all tools should have (Rubright and MacDonald, 1981: 160). For greater productivity, promotional tools should

Reflect marketing and agency objectives and strategies

Be written for specific targets

Carry at least one promotional message

Reflect or suggest service benefit

Reflect organizational purpose

Have a distribution plan

Have acceptable tone, style, and character

Persuade or inform

Be concisely written and edited

Reflect both reader and management needs

Ask for some action or participation by targets

Examples of various promotional tools are given in Table 9.1.

In evaluating which media to use, Weinrauch (1987) states the advantages and disadvantages of several types of media, as summarized in Table 9.2. This summary should assist the administrator in choosing media for the agency's promotional campaign. Some of the other promotional tools are highlighted in more detail in the following sections.

Table 9.1 Promotional Tools

Fact sheets	Meetings, seminars, and workshops
Special business letters	Handouts and manuals
Direct mailings	Open houses and tours
Public service announcements	Videotape programs
Comment forms from clients	News conferences or releases
Questionnaires and surveys	Regional and local magazines
Displays, fairs, and exhibits	Posters
Information racks	Coupons
Bulletin boards	Annual reports
Films and audiovisual items	Billboards
Speaker's bureaus	Contests
Feature stories	Signs and graphics
Inserts and enclosures in mailings	Telephone hotlines
Local cable television	Personal selling
Skywriting	Directories
Journals	Transit signs
Home parties	Novelty items
Newsletters	Business cards
Television ads	Radio ads
Health education	Awards

Table 9.2 Advantages and Disadvantages of Specific Promotional Tools

Tools	Advantages	Disadvantages
Television	Reaches large/select audience	Has only partial audience selectivity
	Combines sight, sound, and motion	Has high cost
	Gives opportunities for creative demonstration	Commercial production requirements are high
	Is geographically selective	Message has short life
	Program may be national	Ad must compete with others in short time period
		Frequent repeat is necessary
Radio	Reaches large/selective audience	Is less attention getting than TV
	Is personal and intimate	Appeals to only one sense
	Is immediate and flexible	Message has short life
		Background sound competes

Table 9.2 (*Continued*)

Tools	Advantages	Disadvantages
Radio (*Continued*)	Has low cost (per unit of time) Is usually local Has mass use Uses music	Ad must compete with others in short time period Frequent repeat is necessary
Newspaper	Has low cost Advertiser can make short-term commitment Is flexible and timely Printed word has high believability Is geographically selective Reaches large/selective audience	Offers limited color Lacks secondary readership Has short life Has poor-quality reproduction Is read hastily
Magazine	Provides market segmentation Allows good color Has prestige Has long life Has secondary readership Offers quality reproduction	Audience build-up is slow Lacks flexibility Has long closing dates Is more expensive than newspaper Has waste circulation Offers no guarantee of ad position unless premium paid in advance
Direct mail	Offers audience selectivity Is personal Is flexible No other ads compete Is speedy Is likely to be kept/posted Has special uses Variety of formats is available	Has high cost per reader Gets little attention Throw-away factor is high Mailing lists may not be up to date
Billboard	Is flexible Has impact Competing ads relatively absent Has low cost Has large size Offers repeat exposure	Is open to public attack (ecological implications) Offers no audience selectivity Must be seen quickly Has creative limitations/brief message Viewer has many distractions

Source: Weinrauch, D. *The Marketing Problem Solver.* Copyright © 1987 by John Wiley & Sons, Inc. Reprinted by permission of John Wiley & Sons, Inc.

Brochures

The most common tool is the agency brochure. The agency can use brochures to get its message across to a variety of clients. In addition to the guidelines already given on how to develop a good message, here is some additional information on what should be detailed in the brochure (Rubright and MacDonald, 1981: 162–163):

1. What are the purposes of the organization?
2. What services are offered?
3. What benefits do services provide to targets?
4. How do potential clients make initial contact with the agency?
5. Who do prospective clients first talk with on their initial visit or contact with the agency?
6. Who uses the agency's services?
7. What is the typical routine for the average user of the agency services?
8. How do clients pay for the agency's services?
9. When are agency services available?
10. What routine follow-up or referral is practiced by agency staff?
11. What constitutes the agency's professional staff?
12. How is the agency managed and governed?
13. Where is the agency located?
14. Which organizations certify or accredit the agency?
15. What key memberships does the agency hold?
16. Does the artwork or photographs depict typical clients using agency services?

News Releases

The news release is mailed or distributed by the agency on its letterhead to all communications media, including newspapers, radio, television, and journals. Consideration should be given to deadlines of the various media. A card file should be kept on all media, and the deadlines should be recorded on the cards. Releases are usually used to inform people of a current situation or future development.

Health Fairs

Health Screenings or educational fairs can be conducted to increase people's awareness of health. Often agencies are asked to participate by having a booth at such health fairs. This tool is useful as part of a public awareness campaign. For information on planning health fairs, see the following articles:

Blumenthal, D., Kahn, H., Planning a community health fair. *Public Health Reports.* 94(March/April 1979):156–161.

Germer, P., Price, J. Organization and evaluation of health fairs. *Journal of School Health.* 51(February 1981):86–90.

Mason, D. J., Calvaca, L. R. Health fair: providing a learning experience through a community service project. *Journal of Nursing Education.* 21(June 1982):39–47.

Richie, N. Some guidelines for conducting a health fair. *Public Health Reports.* 91(May/June 1976):261–264.

Watkins, A. How about a health fair. *Pediatric Nursing.* (March/April 1983):123–125.

Watts, P., Stinson, W. The health education carnival. *Health Education.* 12(November/December 1981):23–25.

Watts, P., Stinson, W. Health fairs are more than a community relations scheme; they save dollars and detect health problems early. *Cost Containment.* 5(July 26, 1983):1–2.

Videotapes

Increasingly, videotapes are becoming a major means of communicating with the public. This tool constitutes an excellent means of informing the public on issues. Various organizations produce tapes on care in the home, what home care is, and specific procedures for the family care giver to follow. Agencies can purchase these tapes or develop their own. Many purchased videotapes can be customized by putting the agency's name, address, and phone number at the end.

Some sources of videos on home health care are the following:

Health Care Concepts
27665 Off Bradley Rd.
Lake Forest, IL 60045

Video Library
National Association for Home Care
519 C Street NE
Washington, DC 20002

National In-Home Health Services
14549 Archwood St.
Van Nuys, CA 91405

Healthcare Concepts, Inc.
633 Monroe Ave.
Memphis, TN 38103

Foster Medical Corporation
Home Health Care Division
1000 Conshohocken Rd.
Conshohocken, PA 19428

Hospital Home Health Care Agency of California
23456 Hawthorne Blvd.
Torrance, CA 90505

Seminars, Meetings, and Workshops

Your agency gains credibility among the professionals in home care by conducting seminars, meetings, and workshops. These tools give colleagues a chance to hear the experts in the field discuss issues and solutions. This is also a tool that the agency can use to publicize home care by sending speakers to local AARP meetings, senior citizen centers, church groups, PTAs, and other groups.

Newsletters

One of the newest methods of marketing is the newsletter. Some organizations publish newsletters directed toward clients that your agency can put its name on and send to it clients. An example is *Health at Home*, published by the National Association of Retail Druggists. One issue of this newsletter covered fitness tips, new developments on the health care scene, and information on home diagnostics.

Other newsletters are directed toward professionals in home care. The purpose of all of these newsletters is to educate either the client or the professional. They provide a quick update for families, clients, and professionals on health and the health care field.

Further information about newsletters for the home care industry can be obtained from the following sources:

For the Professional

Home Health Management Advisor
Aspen Publishers
P.O. Box 6018
Gaithersburg, MO 20877

Hospital Home Health
American Health Consultants
Attention: Same-Day Surgery, Dept. 0422
67 Peachtree Park Drive NE
Atlanta, GA 30309

Hospital Product Line
St. Anthony Hospital Publications
P.O. Box 14212
Washington, DC 20077

Health Care Competition Week
Capital Publications
P.O. Box 1454
Alexandria, VA 22313

Physicians Marketing
425 Brannan St.
P.O. Box 77552
San Francisco, CA 94107

Healthcare Advertising Review
1858 Charter Lane
Lancaster, PA 17601

Strategic Health Care Marketing
Health Care Communications
211 Midland Ave.
Rye, NY 10580

High Tech Marketing
1460 Post Road East
Westport, CT 06880

Home Care Economics
American Health Consultants
Home Care Economics Dept. 5398
67 Peachtree Park Drive NE
Atlanta, GA 30309

Healthcare Marketing Report
P.O. Box 76002
Atlanta, GA 30358

Home Health Line
Port Republic, Maryland 20676

Home Health Journal
P.O. Box 19888
Jacksonville, FL 32245

Homecare Clinical Director's Newsletter
c/o National Association for Home Care
519 C Street NE, Stanton Park
Washington, DC 20002

For the Consumer
Health at Home
National Association of Retail Druggists
205 Daingerfield Rd.
Alexandria, VA 22314

Magazines

Another new tool is the magazine directed toward the consumer. One such magazine is *Home Care Consumer,* written exclusively for home care patients. It addresses their concerns for quality of life and wellness. Again, a space is left on the front cover for your agency's name. Further information about this magazine may be obtained from

Home Care Consumer
550 Frontage Rd.
Northfield, IL 60093

Such prepared newsletters and magazines constitute a cost-effective way for an agency to use a professionally produced publication as if it was their own.

Home Parties

St. Elizabeth's Medical Center in Dayton, Ohio, came up with the idea of at-home health parties (Blumenshield, 1986). Its Body Cues program has served over 2,000 women in 2 years and strives to teach women more about their bodies.

The woman who hosts the party receives printed invitations to send to her friends, and the medical center furnishes party materials and game prizes. The 2-hour parties begin with a game in which participants pass around a doctor's black bag containing instruments used during examinations. Each instrument is explained, as is the examination procedure. There is also a discussion on pelvic exams, mammograms, and how to perform breast self-examination. Currently, the program has four to five parties per month.

If one marketing objective is to increase awareness of your agency, this is a fairly low-cost way of becoming more visible as well as teaching people about their health. Topics can be varied to meet the audience's needs.

Further information about health house parties can be obtained from

Body Cues Manager
St. Elizabeth's Corporations
601 Edwin C. Moses Blvd.
Dayton, OH 45408.

CONCLUSION

Promotion is communication that tells potential users about an agency's services. In marketing, promotional tools carry direct messages to targets. These messages are funneled through four channels: advertising, personal selling, public relations, and incentives.

Whatever channel is used, communication requires a source, a message, a means of transmitting the message, and a receiver. Developing the message for the receiver involves tailoring the message for the various channels.

Each message has a grabber, theme, body, hook, and signature. These parts make up the total message of the agency and address the predetermined marketing objective.

A variety of promotional tools can carry the message to the public. Brochures, news releases, health fairs, videotapes, seminars, newsletters, magazines, and home parties are examples of such tools.

Promotional tools are part of every agency's marketing plan. Consideration must be given to what channel and tools should be used to reach the target audience. All of this is done through good assessment of the target population and using the media that will best match their interest.

REFERENCES

Assael, H. *Consumer Behavior and Marketing Action.* Boston: Kent, 1984.

Blumenshield, P. Doctors and nurses promote health in party setting. *Health Link.* 3(September 1986):51.

Chapman, A. (ed.). Developing a new logo or slogan. *Home Care Marketer.* 1(September 1985):2, 6.

Crompton, J., Lamb, C. *Marketing Government and Social Services.* New York: John Wiley & Sons, 1986.

Kotler, P. *Marketing for Nonprofit Organizations* (2nd ed.). Englewood Cliffs, NJ: Prentice-Hall, 1982.

MacLachlan, J., Making a message memorable and persuasive. *Journal of Advertising Research.* 23(December 1983/January 1984):51.

MacStravic, R. *Managing Health Care Marketing Communications.* Rockville, MD: Aspen, 1986.

Rubright, R., MacDonald, D. *Marketing Health and Human Services.* Rockville, MD: Aspen, 1981.

Weinrauch, J. D. *The Marketing Problem Solver.* New York: John Wiley & Sons, 1987.

10

Professional
Personal Selling

Personal selling is the most obvious part of the marketing mix. This chapter discusses personal selling as part of a home health care agency's marketing mix. The five types of salespeople are identified, and the two most useful to home health care agencies are elaborated. Guidelines on how to prepare for and conduct professional personal sales calls are also presented.

As discussed in Chapter 1, the marketing mix consists of at least four Ps, one of which is promotion. Personal selling is a part of promotion, along with public relations, sales promotion (incentives), and advertising. When all the promotional tools are used together in a coordinated fashion, they are "somewhat interchangeable and are synergistic" (Petit and McEnally, 1985:42). Personal selling is the most obvious part of the marketing mix, in part because more money is spent on personal selling than any other aspect of marketing, including advertising (Kotler, 1984). Personal selling is considered most effective when used with organizational (institutional) buyers and when negotiation and/or explanation is necessary to complete the buying process. Because personal selling is expensive, it is most cost effective when a limited number of potential contacts exist, such as hospital discharge planners and medical doctors who are likely to write orders for home health care, or when specific consumer prospects have indicated an interest through responses to advertisements, inquiries, and so on.

Personal selling should have a significant role in marketing home health care. First, home health care serves a variety of publics (e.g., individuals, discharge planners, and medical doctors), all of whom have different needs that home health care can meet. To tailor advertising messages to each of these target markets would be inefficient and prohibitively expensive. Personal selling allows the home health agency to customize its offering and message to meet each of its prospective client's needs. Second, home health care is an intangible service. Personal selling helps explain the benefits of a service that cannot be seen or touched. Also, personal selling is critical in establishing an agency's professional image, which reflects on the quality of care given. Third, personal selling establishes a rapport between the agency, the decision maker, and the client so that if the need arises for additional services, your agency will be thought of first. Finally, personal selling allows for two-way communication and feedback, providing the agency timely information about its services, image, and the marketplace.

If personal selling can provide the home health care agency with all of the benefits just mentioned, why do salespeople have such a bad image? (You would not be the first to associate sales with a person in a plaid jacket, chewed cigar in hand, selling used cars.) It is ironic that those who, in part, are charged with creating, communicating, and maintaining an organization's image have an image problem themselves. Two reasons exist for the bad image of salespeople. One is the human tendency to generalize and stereotype. For instance, most people have an image of a nurse as a female in a white cap and uniform in a hospital setting. As home health care professionals you recognize how inaccurate that image is. That stereotype ignores the significant percentage of nurses who are male, the fact that many hospitals do not require caps and white uniforms, and the fact that a large percentage of nurses are employed outside the hospital setting. Second, the stereotypical image of salespeople is reinforced because of continued exposure to unprofessional sales practices, such as "canned" presentations; salespeople who literally will not take no for an answer; and news stories about unethical atrocities, such as a person being sold aluminum siding for a brick house. In contrast to the erroneous popular image, professional personal selling is an honorable activity for any organization or person.

FIVE TYPES OF PERSONAL SELLING

Different types of personal selling have developed as business has developed and changed over the years (see Chapter 1). Traders and merchants predate the industrial revolution. During that time, the only criterion for successful sales was to have goods available. As the industrial revolution spread, merchants adjusted their sales techniques, bringing together a wider variety of goods under one roof, creating the department store. With the advent of improved transportation in the late nineteenth century, peddlers and drummers began traveling the United States, establishing ongoing relationships between producers and retailers (Manning and Reece, 1987). In the twentieth century, the selling era began, when organizations assumed consumers would not buy unless a "substantial effort were made to stimulate interest in products" (Kotler, 1980: 21). This era was characterized by " 'high pressure selling,' manipulation of the buyer, and 'canned' or memorized sales presentations" (Manning and Reece, 1987: 15). As the marketing era began, as early as 1950 in the industrial sector, the role of the salesperson changed to meet the need. This era created the modern salesperson, highly schooled in product and company knowledge; trained to identify and meet the client's needs; and sophisticated in creating and maintaining a professional, quality image.

Each of these historical eras created a personal selling style that exists in certain industries or businesses today. Of course, merchants exist and thrive in the niche of retailing. Peddlers or drummers, now called commercial visitors, survive on personal relationships and conviviality in low-growth, mature, noncompetitive industries where personal relationships, rather than innovations, are valued. The power persuaders grew out of the selling era and exist in sales-oriented businesses today where either the products are considered unsalable (unacceptable) or are indistinguishable from competitors' offerings such that none would be sold were it not for the power of persuasion. The marketing era—in which the focus is on identifying and meeting the clients' needs—has created two "new" types of salespeople: consultative (problem-solving) and partnership (problem preventing). Each of these five types, and their usefulness to the home health care industry, will be discussed in detail.

Of these styles or types, which are useful for home health care marketers? Merchants succeed by existing, promoting their existence, assembling either a wide variety or a specialized selection of products, and attracting prospective clients to their premises. Since home health care services are generally not delivered at your location, this style of personal selling is not appropriate for home health care agencies.

The commercial visitor style cannot be expected to be successful in home health care for two reasons. First, do you want to trust the success of your agency to the charms of your own personality or that of someone you hire, or rely on your own, albeit professional, relationships? (In answer, it would probably be a wiser, safer investment to routinely bet on the seventh horse in the seventh race at any thoroughbred horse track.) Second, two of the three publics that home health care agencies look to for business (discharge planners and medical doctors) do not have time to sit around and chat. They are professionals and should be expected to base their decisions on factors other than personal relationships.

Power persuaders will undoubtedly generate sales revenues in any business in which they participate—for the short term. However, two factors remove this type from serious consideration in home health care. First, power persuaders need not have substantial knowledge about the products or services they sell to be effective, a risky situation when dealing with health care. Second, assuming your agency is in business for the long haul and does not have an unlimited supply of prospective clients, the reputation and image your agency would generate as a result of using those selling methods would be counter-productive, and any success would be short-lived.

The only truly professional personal selling techniques useful and appropriate for home health care agencies are consultative selling (problem-solving) and partnership (problem-preventing) selling.

Consultative selling is providing solutions to problems. Contrasting with less sophisticated forms of selling, consultative selling sees the client as a person [or organization] to be served. Consultative selling is built on a "foundation of authenticity, and emphasizes two-way communication" and "information giving [and gathering], and nego-tiation, rather than manipulation." Consultative selling is a "planned process that involves a minimum of four basic elements: need discovery; selection of the product [service]; need-satisfaction presen-tation; and servicing the sale" (Manning and Reece, 1987: 15).

Consultative selling increases the "personalization, the customer's [client's] participation, and the professionalization of the relation-ship" (Hanah, 1986: 19). To demonstrate how consultative selling differs from other types, think of your last purchase of an automobile. Was the salesperson with whom you dealt trustworthy and profes-sional? Did he or she determine your needs beyond asking how much you wanted to spend? Have you heard from that person since you drove off the lot, even when you were at the dealership getting your car repaired? Most car dealers do not take a consultative selling approach to selling cars. In contrast, suppose you have just purchased an office copier for $10,000, about the price of a small, new car. If the supplier of the copier is professional and competitive, you probably will receive daily phone calls and weekly visits to make sure the copier is working as expected; this activity is designed to meet the needs of your agency.

The second approach is a consultative approach to selling. The same amount of money was spent, both products have about the same expected lifetime, and both products need service to keep functioning properly, yet each dealer uses a very different approach to sales and service. What's the difference? The copier company is using a consul-tative approach; the car dealer is using a power persuasion approach. With which organization would you rather deal? A key to successful sales is to sell the way you like to be sold. Put another way, "When I want to remember how to sell, I simply recall how I—and other people—like to buy" (Johnson et al., 1984: 44).

If consultative selling has a flaw, it is that it is based on the assumption that problems exist. While problems may seem to be a certainty in business, the focus on problems can be negative. Partnership selling, or problem-prevention selling, takes the process of consultative selling one step further, removing the focus on today's problems and concentrating on preventing tomorrow's problems. All the elements of consultative selling are present, but they are future oriented. The differences among the power persuasion, consultative, and partnership approaches are illustrated in Table 10.1.

Because of its orientation toward the future, partnership selling can reasonably be used only by large, established health care agencies— those with enough resources and financial stability to make long-term investments in the future. Partnership selling rewards users with an increased market share and higher future profits in exchange for signing up a client today.

The sales style a home health care agency selects should be based on the agency's culture, financial condition, and philosophy as set forth in its mission statement.

THREE KEYS OF SUCCESSFUL SELLING

Regardless of the selling style an agency chooses, three key rules for successful selling must be followed:

1. Know your client.
2. Know your agency and its services, capabilities, and limitations.
3. Follow up, follow up, follow up.

If these three rules are followed, sales success is virtually guaranteed.

Know Your Client

Think of someone as identical to you as possible—the same age, sex, height, weight, income, education, and career. Do both of you drive identical cars, wear identical clothes, and take vacations to the same places? Probably not, even though the person you thought of was demographically identical to you. Why would that be? The reason is that as individuals we all have different needs regardless how "identical" we may be. As consumers we satisfy those needs in part through our purchases of products and services. Organizations are

Table 10.1   Outcomes of Various Sales Approaches

Selling Approaches	Home Health Care Publics		
	Medical Doctors	Discharge Planners	Prospective Clients
Power persuasion	Case assignment today	Case assignment today	Care given today
Consultative	Agreement to assign patient currently undergoing treatment	Agreement to assign patient currently in hospital	Relationship developed such that when care is needed your agency will be requested
Partnership	Development of total treatment programs for specific conditions, from diagnosis and treatment by doctor, and follow-up and home care by agency	Development of a total care program that involves the agency from the time care is ordered by hospital or sooner	Development of new programs and services that will meet future needs

nothing more than groups of individuals. The organization has needs, just as do the individuals who make up the organization. Since a sale cannot occur until the client perceives that your service will meet his or her needs, knowing your clients and their needs is a crucial first key to sales success.

Two tools are highly useful in developing knowledge of your agency's clients. First, knowing your client requires creative empathy, the ability to put yourself in the other person's shoes. Second, knowing your client requires the ability to listen effectively. The belief of many successful salespeople is that if you listen, prospective clients will tell not only what their needs are, but also how your organization can meet those needs! One key question to ask is, what is your biggest problem (in your situation, with assigning patients to home care, or in dealing with home care agencies)?

The Client as an Individual

The example of an "identical" friend illustrated how two "identical" people can purchase different products or services to meet different needs. Conversely, two different people may purchase the same product or service for very different reasons to meet their very different individual needs. For example, consider the following hypothetical situation. Mr. and Mrs. Smith are living comfortably in their own home. Mrs. Smith is 70 years old and healthy. Mr. Smith, 75 years old, suffers from Alzheimer's disease. Their adult children do not live in the same area but visit as often as possible and are committed to supporting their parents financially if necessary. Because each of the children has a growing family, it is impractical for the Smiths to move in with their adult children. Suggestions from the children that their father be put in a nursing home were rejected because the couple did not want to be separated after 45 years of marriage and because no local nursing homes would accept residents with Alzheimer's disease. One of the couple's sons had recently received home health care following day surgery for appendicitis. As a result of his experience, he suggested to his mother that a home health care service might be able to help her. While his mother was noncommittal to the suggestion, she mentioned it to a friend during a phone conversation. The friend said that last month she had attended a meeting of the local American Association of Retired Persons (AARP), where you had spoken about the variety of services home health care agencies, yours in particular, can provide. As a result, you receive a call from Mrs. Smith. With this scenario, what needs does Mrs. Smith have to be met?

The obvious answer might be, "Mrs. Smith, who is healthy and presumably active, needs her freedom to get out occasionally to see friends or shop. Our homemaker service will allow her to do that." This might be a correct analysis. However, might Mrs. Smith be worried that the care she is giving her husband may not be as good as the care a professional could provide? Therefore, her need might be to have the confidence and knowledge that her husband is receiving the best possible care at home. A different need might be that Mrs. Smith wants to be a better grandmother by being able to visit her grandchildren more frequently. (Note the difference between freedom to do what you *want* and freedom to do what you *should*.) A fourth need of Mrs. Smith's might be to please her children by providing their father with professional care. A fifth need might be the relief of pressure from her children to put their father in a nursing home; this need would be met if she could tell them that he was receiving professional care at home and her burden were eased.

You may be able to identify even more potential needs of Mrs. Smith. The successful salesperson will help Mrs. Smith identify her needs by asking questions such as: What is your problem with the current situation? What would you do if the situation were different? If you could do one activity that this situation prevents you from doing, what would it be? If you could change one thing about your current situation (other than curing your husband's illness), what would it be? Note that these questions are open-ended, encouraging Mrs. Smith to discuss her feelings. Open-ended questions are more effective than closed-end ones, such as, "Wouldn't you rather be going shopping with friends this afternoon?"

Unless you know your client and identify his or her needs, your sales effort will not be successful. If you communicate to Mrs. Smith that she would gain her freedom by utilizing your homemaker services, you will not be successful if she wants to get her children off her back about putting their father in a nursing home.

Knowing your client results from carefully identifying your client's needs. Identifying those needs involves asking open-ended questions and listening to the answers.

The Discharge Planner as a Client

Unlike the clients in the previous example, the discharge planner or a member of his or her family will not be the recipient of your services, will not see the services being delivered, and will not pay for them. Likewise, the discharge planner may not receive immediate feedback as to the satisfactoriness of the services your agency provides. If the discharge planner cannot physically see your services being rendered, then the image of your agency's quality will substitute for first-hand observation (another reason for constantly monitoring, maintaining and improving your agency's image). However, the professional discharge planner will be concerned about the quality of care your agency can provide. If a discharge planner assigns a patient to an agency that provides unsatisfactory care—creating a dissatisfied client—the discharge planner risks the favorable reputation of the hospital where he or she works. Conversely, successful home health care can enhance the image of care provided by the hospital. A need of the discharge planner may be to protect or enhance the hospital's image of quality care.

If the discharge planner is aware of and sensitive to the financial situation of the patient, your agency's price of services may be a factor. If the care of the patient is to be reimbursed by Medicaid-Medicare, then the discharge planner may need to know the status of your agency's Medicaid-Medicare certification. The patient may not be known to the discharge planner personally. In fact, the discharge planner may never have seen the patient or may never see the patient again. The planner's concern about the quality of care the patient receives is determined in part by the planner's attitude toward his or her role in providing the patient care.

Discharge planners' attitudes and needs are also influenced by their attitudes toward their employer and their job. For example, discharge planners are somewhat emotionally, physically, and legally removed from the results of their actions. Conversely, a series of incorrect decisions (or, in the vernacular, foul-ups) may result in the loss of the discharge planner's job. Therefore, one need of a discharge planner might be to do his or her job as well as possible, or to avoid wrong or risky decisions. Likewise, if a hospital has its own home health care agency, the discharge planner's need may be to know what agencies are available to handle overload situations or cases the hospital's agency is not staffed or equipped to handle.

Open-ended questions to ask discharge planners might include: What is the most difficult part of your job as a discharge planner? How does the hospital view your role as a discharge planner? What is the best home health care agency you've assigned a case to? What made that agency the best? Tell me about the worst experience you've had with a home health care agency. What are the most important factors you look for in evaluating a home health care agency?

Again, the needs of the discharge planner differ from person to person, institution to institution, and case to case. Sensitivity to the changeable needs of the discharge planner will help your agency sell your services successfully.

The Medical Doctor as the Client

Currently most home health care consumers are Medicare recipients referred to a home health care agency by a physician (Ponzurick et al., 1987). Ponzurick and coworkers (1987) also found that about 96% of the physicians responding to a survey in the Memphis area had "recommended a home health care agency service to their patients at one time or another." Legg and Lamb (1986: 54) found that "physicians held generally favorable perceptions regarding home health care organizations." However, the physician's role in referring a patient to a home health care agency is similar to the physician's role in prescribing drugs: the prescription is part of the care, but the physician does not receive any financial remuneration for the care prescribed. "Physicians may have little knowledge of what is going on in the home [of a home care patient] yet are held responsible for ordering the care given there—with no reimbursement for doing so" (Mundinger, 1983: 47). While it may be irresponsible to suggest that physicians would only recommend a care plan that would involve reimbursement to their practice, the situation does identify a potential need of physicians for information regarding the patient's progress and care. In addition, it may be in the physician's best interest to recommend home health care if the agency can provide information regarding the patient's condition that may suggest that an office visit is necessary.

For a home health care agency to successfully sell its services to physicians, the agency must recognize that medical doctors are not a homogeneous group. First, medical doctors in specialties such as radiology, anesthesiology, and pathology do not refer patients (Legg and Lamb, 1986). Ponzurick and colleagues (1987) confirmed that 73% of the medical group (podiatry; cardiology; internal medicine; family practice; neurology; obstetrics and gynecology; dermatology; oncology; otology; ear, nose, and throat; endocrinology; urology; and general practice) had recommended the use of a home health care. In comparison, only 11% of the surgical group (thoracic, plastic, general, and orthopedic) and 17% of "nontraditional users" (psychiatry, radiology, genetics, opthalmology, pathology, and anesthesiology) had recommended home health care.

Second, physicians differ in their attitudes toward their practice and home care. Five attitudinal profiles have been suggested: "high tech," "high touch," "care control," "worry relief," and "can't be bothered." (What to say, 1985). Each profile, representing a market segment, has different needs. The high-tech physician, perceiving him- or herself as being "on the cutting edge" of medicine, may tend to focus on an agency's credentials, knowledge of current protocols, standards, and use of high-tech equipment and procedures. The high-touch physician believes in warm, personal care of patients and would expect home health care agencies to exhibit the same attitude. The attitude of care control physicians is that the only good medical care is performed by themselves. Constant feedback to such physicians and documentation that *their* care plan is being implemented will help meet their needs. Similar to the care control physician is the doctor with the worry relief profile. Worry relief physicians worry about the quality of care in the "uncontrolled" environment of the home as well as about responsibility, accountability, and liability for themselves and the home health care agency.

The can't be bothered physicians want one-stop shopping. Your agency's ability to provide *all* home care services will meet this group's needs.

Questions that will help identify the physician's profile and needs regarding home health care might be: What role should a home health agency play in the treatment plan for your patients? What has been your most successful experience with a home health agency? What has been your biggest problem in working with home health agencies? How do you recognize a good home health care agency?

Utilizing physician profiles to help identify and meet the physician's needs is not as simple as asking, What kind of a physician are you? Correctly categorizing a physician according to a certain profile does not guarantee sales success. The profiles described here are tools to guide your thinking in identifying and meeting the physician's needs.

Know Your Agency

Just as knowing your client focuses on information gathering, knowing your agency focuses on information giving. The professional salesperson is a bona fide source of information. After all, who knows more about an agency's services and capabilities than the marketer or administrator? Therefore, an important part of successful selling is informing prospective clients about the benefits the agency's services offer and how those services might meet the client's needs.

Knowing the services and capabilities of your agency increases the agency's value to the client and the professional image of the agency. Knowledge of those services "builds confidence in one's abilities, and helps in meeting objectives" (Anderson, 1987: 92-93). The quality of care in the agency is reflected in the agency's image. Nothing affects an agency's image more than the professionalism of the personnel making sales contacts. One very important factor in creating a professional image is being knowledgeable about the agency's services and capabilities. A sales call occupies the prospective client's time. How you feel when a person has wasted your time? More often than not, that time was wasted when the person to whom you were talking provided no information that you did not already know or provided information that did not meet your current needs. Knowing the services and capabilities of your agency will help keep you from wasting a client's time. Implied in the definition of a professional is that he or she is knowledgeable enough about a subject to be paid for that information.

Being a professional salesperson takes confidence in the services and capabilities of your agency as well as confidence in your own abilities. (Other factors that create and motivate people to sell are discussed later.)

A weight lifter developing muscles is building confidence in his or her ability to lift heavier weights. Similarly, learning and knowing more about your agency's services and capabilities builds your confidence in being able to identify and meet clients' needs.

Yes is the word a salesperson loves to hear. However, no is heard much more frequently. Although several ways of dealing with objections are discussed later, one of the best defenses against objections is knowledge of your services. You lose an opportunity to gain a client or close a sale when you say "I don't know" or "Can I get back to you on that?" Knowledge of your agency reduces the need to give such responses. However, you should *never, never lie.* "I don't know" or "Can I get back to you on that?" is *always* better and more professional than a guess or an outright lie!

Follow Up, Follow Up, Follow Up

The third key concept in successful professional selling is following up. Knowledge of your agency may reduce the frequency of responding with "I don't know" and "Can I get back to you on that?"; however, when the client's questions cannot be answered, another opportunity exists for the professional salesperson to enhance his or her professional image and that of the agency. Telling a client, "I can have that information for you on Thursday," is making a promise. There is no difference between promising information on Thursday and promising to provide home care to a client. Both are promises. Clients tend to believe that irresponsibility in little things indicates irresponsibility in all things. Following up thoroughly is as simple as taking notes during sales calls and telephone conversations coupled with keeping a calendar.

For example, during a telephone conversation on Monday with a discharge planner from Memorial Hospital, you are asked, "Can you begin infusion therapy on a client this Thursday?" Because you cannot predict what your client load will be next Thursday, you may have to say, "I can't say today, but I'll know for sure on Wednesday morning. Will it meet your need if I call you with the information on Wednesday, first thing?" Assuming you receive an affirmative answer, make a note on tomorrow's (Tuesday's) calendar: "11:00 A.M. check work load infusion therapist for Mem. Hosp.," and on Wednesday's calendar write "# 1. Call Mem. Hosp. re: inf. ther." Making such notes immediately virtually ensures that, regardless of how hectic your days become, you will be reminded to follow up.

Following up is a trait of a professional salesperson representing a professional organization. To examine a more problematic example of professionalism, let us take the previous example one step further. Late Tuesday afternoon, reminded by your calendar notes, you discover that your agency cannot handle the case starting Thursday. What do you do?

The worst action you could take would be to do nothing, not even informing the discharge planner of the situation. This "ostrich" technique is totally unprofessional and irresponsible. Using such a technique will destroy any professional image you have worked to achieve and severely damage your relationship with that discharge planner. Perhaps the best, most professional approach would be to call the discharge planner *as soon as* you have the information, saying, "I was checking our work load in preparation for calling you tomorrow morning and I discovered that—as much as I hate saying it— we are unable to accept another infusion therapy patient starting Thursday. Is the patient you were thinking of assigning to us still scheduled to be discharged Thursday?" (You are determining if the situation has changed to an extent where you might be able to handle this case.) If the answer is, "No the patient won't be discharged until Monday," ask for the opportunity to check back later in the week. If the answer is, "Yes, the patient will be discharged Thursday," the most professional thing to say is, "I sincerely regret we can't take this case, and I sincerely thank you for the opportunity. I've done some checking, and I know that competitor B would be able to take this case starting Thursday. I hope that this information may be of some help. Will you please consider us on the next case where we can help?"

This example may be surprising—even shocking—to some people. Obviously, one cannot run an ongoing business by continually referring clients to competitors. However, this example illustrates a professional, long-term sales approach.

First, by facing up to the situation, you have demonstrated that you have a responsible agency. Second, by calling (or even trying to call) before the expected time you have shown respect for the discharge planner and an understanding of his or her job. Third, by asking if the situation has changed, you are rechecking to see if an opportunity for your agency still exists and are demonstrating an understanding that a discharge planner's job is constantly changing. Fourth, by informing the discharge planner that competitor B can take the case, you have provided the discharge planner with a solution, rather than a problem: (Remember that Consultative selling is problem-solving selling.) You have made the discharge planner's job easier. Fifth, the discharge planner will later recall this incident in a positive light because you helped solve a problem, rather than in a negative light, remembering only that your agency was unable to handle a case. Finally, you took the opportunity to ask that your agency be considered for the next opportunity. In sales jargon, that is called asking for the order, a very important part of the sales call.

THE SALES CALL

Making a successful sales call is more than popping your head into a physician's office and asking, "You don't have any patients to assign to home health care today, do you?" That approach probably met with little success when you were 10 years old and selling band candy or Scout cookies, and it will certainly meet with less success if you are selling home health care. There is more to a sales to call than what goes on in the prospective client's office. The professional sales call consists of five parts: preparation, opening, building interest and desire, closing, and follow-up.

Preparation

Preparation includes everything one does before walking into a prospective client's office. The first step in preparation is identifying prospective clients. As a result of the agency's mission statement, objectives, and market audit, you should have a clear idea as to what the agency's target markets are. Identifying prospects is determining the individuals and organizations that make up target markets. Prospecting also includes finding the names of prospective contacts. This can be done by using mailing lists and membership lists from professional or interest organizations, or calling a hospital and asking for the name of the discharge planner. In addition, some research can be done on the client or client's organization to anticipate what the client's needs may be. However, do not let your anticipation of clients' needs close your mind to what the clients will identify as their needs!

The second part of preparation is planning the actual sales call.

First, what is the objective—the desired outcome—of this contact? It is to develop information about the client's needs? Is it to sign up a case? Is it to introduce the client to your agency? Setting an objective for the call greatly influences how the sales call is conducted.

The third part of the preparation is a sales call checklist, shown in Table 10.2. The sales call checklist is a convenient tool to help ensure efficient, professional sales calls. The first item on the list reminds the salesperson to review the expected contact's name and title. Remember that clients' days do not always go according to plan and that clients' schedules can change unexpectedly; therefore, have an alternative person's name you wish to see should the prime prospect be unavailable.

Next, double-check the appointment time. Making sure that the appointment is for 10:30 rather than 10:00 will avoid wasting time waiting. Conversely, arriving at 10:30 for a 10:00 appointment is unprofessional and adversely effects the client's image of the salesperson and the agency he or she represents.

Review the location. One usually professional salesperson expected to meet a new client at Seventy-second Street and Harvard, which turned out to be an empty field. This person's client was at Seventy-second Street and South Harvard, 15 miles away. Rechecking the address avoids embarrassing problems such as this. Also, rechecking the address allows the salesperson to leave time for such location-dependent activities as finding a parking place.

Make sure your objectives are established. A professional salesper-

Table 10.2 Sales Call Checklist

☐ Whom I will be seeing. Title. Alternative, if unavailable.
☐ Check appointment time.
☐ Review location, including directions, if necessary.
☐ Establish objectives for call.
☐ Review previous contacts, if any.
☐ Double-check for uncompleted follow-up items.
☐ Think of client's nonbusiness interests.
☐ Check "take with" items.
    ☐ Business cards
    ☐ Brochures and agency information
    ☐ Promotional items (pens, memo pads, etc.)
    ☐ Pricing information
    ☐ Your own pen and notebook

---

son never sees a client without having a purpose or objective for the visit.

Review previous contacts. What has been discussed in previous contacts? Are there unresolved issues? Were needs identified that have not been fully investigated?

Double-check for uncompleted follow-up items. Were promises of action or information made that have yet to be accomplished? Professionalism suffers when the client asks, "Did you bring the information I requested on your agency's case management services?" and the salesperson responds, "Oops, I forgot."

Think of the client's nonbusiness interests. Depending on the client's personal style, time pressures, and job, some sales calls may be 100% business, and others—even with the same client—might involve a significant portion of nonbusiness topics. Think of what topics the client enjoys discussing, such as children, hobbies, or sports.

Finally, check "take with" items. Professional salespeople always have their own pen and paper, an adequate supply of business cards, agency information and brochures, promotional items, and pricing information.

When making a sales call or even just prospecting, it is usually best to have an appointment. Appointments have several advantages. Making appointments can save time because you can expect to see a person at the stated time. Appointments support the professional, businesslike image you have for your agency. The client feels important because you took the time to schedule a call, as opposed to dropping in. Having an appointment assures a more receptive attitude and allows the client to prepare for your visit, both of which can result in more productive sales calls. In addition, setting up the appointment can provide the opportunity to develop background information on the client and start the process of identifying the client's needs.

The opposite of making calls with an appointment is cold calling or dropping in. Cold calling or dropping in can create an unfavorable impression. If you were to say, "I was in the area, so I thought I'd stop by to tell you about our home care services," the client may interpret that as, "What? The only reason you came to see me was because you were in the area? You're telling me that I'm not important enough to you to come by and see me on purpose!" A negative first impression is not the best way to start a sales call or a business relationship.

However, cold calls have some advantages. They are quick, convenient, economical, productive, and flexible. Cold calls can be a good way to initially qualify prospects. Cold calls can also be used to fill time when an appointment is canceled or a scheduled sales call is completed in less time than you had anticipated.

Regardless of the advantages or disadvantages of appointments versus cold calls, clients will inform a salesperson which method they prefer. (If they don't, ask.) Doctors may set aside a particular time in the week when they will see any salesperson in their office. Some doctors may see only those who have an appointment during the time set aside. Some may accept appointments only the week of the call; others, not less than a week in advance. The same is true for discharge planners. Determining and complying with clients' preferences regarding appointments is another way of identifying and meeting clients' needs.

Telephone Etiquette

The telephone has become a powerful business tool. Whether you are calling to set up an appointment, following up on a previous personal call, or reviewing case information, several rules of telephone etiquette can help make your conversation more productive. These rules are outlined in Table 10.3.

The first rule is always smile, assuming the subject is not death. Although a telephone seems to be only an auditory device, smiles can

Table 10.3   Rules of Telephone Etiquette

1. Always smile.
2. Be pleasant.
3. Respect the person who answers the phone.
4. Ask for names and their correct spellings.
5. If making an appointment, be prepared to give a full sales presentation.
6. Do
   Talk distinctly and directly into the mouthpiece.
   Pay attention.
   Set objectives for the phone call.
   If making an appointment, have alternative times or dates available.
   Keep control of the call.
7. Don't
   Smoke.
   Shuffle papers.
   Cradle the phone on your shoulder.
   Take another call.

be seen and frowns can be heard. Smiling pleasantly while talking on the phone automatically makes one's voice more pleasant and one's tone more positive.

Always be pleasant. Never use innuendos or make facetious remarks. Because your facial expressions, such as a raised eyebrow or a wink, cannot be seen, everything said will be taken literally. Likewise, show respect to whomever answers the phone. First, many organizations have a policy that everybody answers their own phone, so the person who answers may be the person you want to see. Second, the caller has no way of knowing the role the person who answers the phone may play in the decision making process. To your chagrin, you may discover that the person you thought was "only a secretary" is the person who writes the orders for the discharge planner's approval.

Finally, if the purpose of the phone call is to arrange an appointment, have alternative dates and times in mind so that that purpose can be accomplished without having to call back. Also, be prepared to conduct the sales presentation. If one receives the response, "I can't see you Thursday, but I have some time to talk on the phone now," what should you do? If you are prepared, you can take advantage of the opportunity. However, depending on the purpose of the call, deferring business until a personal visit may be the best alternative.

Roles in the Buying Decision

Anyone selling to organizations must recognize the various roles potential clients play in the decision-making process. Of course, the people have titles, such as receptionist, discharge planner, outpatient services administrator, and so on. However, the title one person has may be misleading as to their actual role in the decision-making process. Complicating the selling process, one person may play more than one role. Since each role has a different function in the decision-making process and each role entails different needs, the astute salesperson must understand the roles and recognize the needs of each.

The six roles found in the decision-making process are initiator, influencer, decision maker, buyer, user, and gatekeeper, as defined in Table 10.4.

To understand how various people in groups can take on these roles in the decision process, consider the following example. You, the salesperson of XYZ Agency, are in the lobby of Memorial Hospital waiting to see J. Smith, the supervisor of discharge planning services. XYZ Agency has never had a referral from Memorial. The objectives of

Table 10.4   Roles in the Decision-making Process

Initiator	Person or group that first recognizes a need for your agency's services or sees that a problem can be solved with home health care
Influencer	Person or group whose opinions are valued or required, formally or informally, in the decision-making process
Decision maker	Person (rarely a group) who has the formal authority and/or informal power to make the final decision
Buyer	Person who actually carries out the formal process of assigning or contracting for home care services
User	Clients, those who actually are the recipients of home health care services
Gatekeeper	Anyone or group within the organization that controls the flow of information to others in the organization who are a part of the decision-making process.

the sales call are to determine why XYZ Agency has not received referrals and to review with J. Smith the newest of XYZ's services: high-tech care for premature infants. While you are waiting, you see B. Jones, an acquaintance who is an accountant with the hospital. After exchanging greetings Jones says, "I'd love to talk, but I've got to run. The chief administrator wants a report from me, like yesterday!" You ask, "What's up?" Jones says, "Last week, one of my analyses showed that we're losing money on every premature infant we have in the place, because of prospective payments. And now I have to do a detailed analysis—by noon!" You ask, "Are you assigning any of those babies to home care?" "Huh? Uh—I don't know. Why?" says Jones. You say, "You might be able to reduce some of those babies' time in the hospital if they were taken home and provided home health care." Jones says, heading down the hall, "Gee, I don't know. Sounds interesting. Maybe we'll talk sometime, but I've got to get to this report. That administrator wants solutions!" The next day while discussing the report with the chief administrator, Jones says, "I don't have any numbers on this, but have we looked into home health care for 'preemies'?"

Shortly after "Jones" goes down the hall you're in Smith's office. Smith is saying, "The reason your agency hasn't received any cases is that you are not on our approved list. I decide to whom we assign cases, but the Agency Approval Committee must approve any agency before we assign any cases. I sit on the committee along with the chief administrator, the head of nursing, the chief medical officer, and one of our social workers. Until you're approved, there's nothing I can do."

What roles did you see in this scenario? Do you think your agency will receive referrals?

First, who is the decision maker? Ultimately, the decision maker is the key person, the one who will decide to assign your agency a case. In the example, Smith is the ultimate decision maker; Smith will eventually decide whether or not to utilize your agency's services. However, even if you are able to meet all of Smith's needs, you will not automatically be assigned cases because of the influential role of the Agency Approval Committee. While that group does not decide which agency will get which patients, meeting that group's needs is critical to receiving cases. Therefore, their needs must be met first.

Who was the initiator? In one sense you were, initiating the process to receive cases. On the other hand, your acquaintance Jones acted as initiator by discussing home care with the chief administrator as a solution to a problem. While Jones is not in a position to determine or even influence your eventual case load from this hospital, Jones's activities may have a significant impact on your agency's image as a creative problem solver with this hospital. Also, notice that in your conversation with Jones you focused on a problem solution ("Home health care may help") rather than on self-promotion ("Our agency handles preemies all the time.")

What could be the outcome of this scenario? Ideally, the chief administrator will take on the role of initiator and call Smith, asking about home health care for premature infants. Smith might respond, "I was talking with an agency about exactly that earlier today. But this agency hasn't been approved by the committee." (Note that Smith is now in the role of gatekeeper—controlling information—since Smith could just as easily have said, "No, that's not possible. None of our approved agencies do that.") The administrator might say, "Let's get the committee together as soon as possible and get those people in to tell us what they can do. Maybe we can kill two birds with one stone—solve a problem and approve that agency all at one meeting." The end result is that you make your presentation, obtain the committee's approval, solve the administrator's problem, and make the discharge planner look good for finding a solution; and, of course, your agency has begun a long and profitable relationship with Memorial Hospital.

This scenario is idealized, complete with a perfect, happy ending. However, it serves to illustrate how roles in the decision-making process can change and how the same people can play different roles and have different needs.

More about Gatekeepers. The role of gatekeeper is one of the most powerful in the decision-making process, second only to that of decision-maker. (What would have happened in the example if Smith had told the administrator that home health care was not a solution because none of the approved agencies could provide it?) Unfortunately, people do not wear signs saying "gatekeeper." Gatekeepers can be found in virtually any situation and any job description. Receptionists, secretaries, and telephone operators routinely function as gatekeepers by passing along or discarding the information you leave, or providing unofficial information about the decision maker, business conditions, or your competitors. Physicians can be gatekeepers by deciding whether to discuss home care options with patients and colleagues.

Users. Users, or clients, can also play a role in the decision-making process. Their power to refuse care can have an impact on your business. The users' power to provide feedback to the decision maker on the quality of care given may strongly influence your success in getting additional referrals. The power of word-of-mouth advertising that users can generate was discussed in Chapter 2.

Knowing the roles people play in the decision-making process can help you identify their individual and organizational needs. Understanding the roles can help your home health agency understand the process by which decisions to use your agency are made.

ANATOMY OF A SALES CALL

Any point in promotion—including personal selling—must include the four steps represented by the acronym AIDA: attention, interest, desire, and action (McDaniel and Darden, 1987). For personal selling, AIDA translates into opening, building interest and desire, closing, and follow-up.

Opening

You have only one chance to make a good first impression. First impressions are made up of what you do and say and how you appear.

Your first impression with a client starts when the appointment is set up or even before the first contact, as a result of your agency's image. When you first meet someone, that person begins forming a first impression based on what he or she can see. Based on research (Elsea, 1984: 10), the order in which impressions are processed and retained is:

Color of skin

Gender

Age

Appearance

Facial expressions

Eye contact

Movement (smooth/clumsy)

Personal space

Touch

If this list appears to reinforce unfavorable stereotypes, do not be alarmed. This list is only what people remember based on first impressions. Contrast the list with the one in Table 10.5, which was adapted from research done by the Whirlpool Corporation to determine the important characteristics of a salesperson. The difference between the two lists is that the first reflects what people remember about a first impression and the second reflects the characteristics of the person with whom they want to do business.

Remember that visual first impressions include how you dress. From the way you dress people infer the level of your education, income, sophistication, your trustworthiness, and even your moral character (Thourlby, 1980). While different parts of the United States have different standards of acceptable business dress, generally speaking your dress should be conservative, appropriate to the occasion, simple, and of the highest quality affordable. To "dress for success," a term coined by Molloy (1975, 1977, 1981), always check your appearance in a mirror—even the car's rearview mirror—before making a sales call.

First impressions are created not only by how you look but also by how you sound, what you say, and how well you listen (Elsea, 1984). Your voice reflects your stress level and level of fatigue. Your voice is characterized by the rate of speaking, volume, pitch, timbre (or

Table 10.5   Important Characteristics of a Salesperson

Characteristic	Percent Responding "Always Important"
Courteous	91
Knowledgeable about services, company	72
Knowledgeable about competition	39
Available	37
The same sex as you	6
The same ethnic background as you	3
The same age as you	2

Source: Manning, G. L., Reece, B. L. *Selling Today: A Personal Approach* (3rd ed.). Dubuque, IA: William C. Brown, 1987.

quality), and articulation. The proper level of your speaking rate, volume, pitch, and timbre vary according to the situation, for example, with whether you are addressing a large meeting or talking across a desk to one person. The only way to judge your own voice is to hear an audio recording of it and to practice relaxing as you speak. The use of habitual filler phrases, such as "you know"; colloquialisms, such as "youse" or "gonna;" and mispronounciations, such as "git" for "get" and "fil-um" for "film" is not only distracting but also detracts from your professional image. Most important, your voice should communicate the confidence and enthusiasm you have for your agency, its services, and yourself.

What to say to open a sales call is determined by each particular situation. Your relationship with the contact, the contact's and your own time constraints, and the contact's and your personality will determine whether it is more effective to chat about general or personal items and then get down to business or to be strictly business.

Building Interest and Desire

Building interest and desire is the part of the sales call in which you identify the client's needs and determine how your agency's services can best meet those needs first-hand. Whenever possible, ask open-ended questions. Ask, "What home health care services are you currently using?" (open ended) rather than "Do you use home health care services?" (yes/no). One way of identifying opportunities is ask prospective clients what they have and then what they want (Johnson and Wilson, 1984). The difference between the two is the opportunity: the need that your agency may be able to fill.

Benefits versus Features
Benefits are what an agency can do for a client or decision maker (or someone playing any of the other five roles). Features are facts about your services and agency. Put another way, features are what sales-people brag about, and benefits are the reason decision makers buy. For example, a feature of a car is that it gets 30 miles per gallon. The benefits of getting 30 miles per gallon could be that you will save money because the car uses little gas or that you will have more time to do important things because you will not have to stop for gas as often.

The benefits of a feature are easier to determine when you have identified and understand the client's needs. For example, a feature of a particular home health care agency might be that it is able to provide care 24 hours a day. The potential benefit of that feature to discharge planners might be the confidence of doing their job better because there will be no complaints about lapses in care. For physicians the benefit may be similar or may be that they will be able to provide better care because the patient can be observed 24 hours a day. For the client, the benefit would be peace of mind knowing that care is available anytime that care is needed.

Handling Objections
Frequently in discussing how the services an agency offers might meet the client's needs, sales resistance—objections—are encountered. When an objection, usually characterized by the word no, is encountered, it should be dealt with immediately, otherwise, the client will assume that you have accepted the objection. Objections can be feedback showing that the prospect does not understand the benefits of the service.

Sales resistance can stem from a variety of causes and can be dealt with in a variety of ways. If the prospect has a fear of change, assurance will ease that fear. If the prospect is unfamiliar with one's agency or services, the solution is education. With experience, the professional salesperson will be able to anticipate sales resistance and be prepared to discuss the client's objections successfully.

When an objection is encountered, restate the objection. This allows you to demonstrate an understanding of the problem. Restating the objection enables the salesperson to isolate the objection from other considerations. Ask questions to better understand the problem. Find some point of agreement. Never argue with the prospect. Never ask the prospect to change his or her mind; rather, provide additional information so that the prospect can make a new decision!

Closing

A sale is made when the client "gets the maximum benefits with the minimum personal risk" (Johnson and Wilson, 1984: 61). At some point in your presentation you must close the sale. Simply put, this means asking for a particular action or asking for the order. Closing also means asking the client to take the action that will achieve your goals and objectives for the call.

Clients give closing cues when they have convinced—that is, sold—themselves on the value of your services. The least subtle closing cue is a direct question: "Can you start with this case today?" Positive statements about your services or agency may be closing clues, or a restatement of benefits may indicate which benefits are particularly important to the client.

When you receive cues indicating agreement, *ask for the desired action.* Ask directly, "Will you assign us your next case?" Other closing methods include eliminating the single objection (e.g., "When we document our Medicare certificate, will we be assigned your next case?") and limited choice closing ("Would you anticipate assigning us a case Thursday or Friday?") (Manning and Reece, 1987).

Finally, when you get the order—that is, achieve the objective or goal, always say thank you. Restate the action the client is expected to take and the action the agency will take. When those actions are confirmed, leave. The client is a busy person with other important things to do. As the salesperson, you have accomplished your objective, so there is no need to stay.

Follow-up

The importance of following up was discussed earlier. After a sales call, follow up with a letter confirming the discussion. Be sure to address any unanswered objections or questions.

FINAL WORDS ON SELLING

Successful salespeople are eternal optimists. They honestly believe in their agency and its services. Their attitude when a prospect rejects their offering is that the only reason could be that the benefits were not explained properly. In other words, they think, "Nobody in their right mind could utilize an agency other than mine."

The last word on professional selling is *never knock the competition.* Knocking the competition is unprofessional and counterproductive. Would you prefer to gain clients because your agency has the highest quality, best value, and service or because all the other agencies are worse than yours?

SELECTION OF SALESPEOPLE

When a home health care agency decides to use personal selling as part of its marketing mix, the decision as to who will be responsible for personal sales can be problematical, as can the selection of those who will have the sales responsibility. In part, the determination of who will have sales responsibility will be influenced by factors such as the size of the agency, plans for growth, makeup of the population of potential and established clients, competitors' actions regarding sales, and the owner's or manager's attitude toward sales. Obviously, a large agency would be more likely to be able to support a full-time sales professional. A smaller agency may find it more advantageous to provide sales training to professional employees, allowing more efficient use of slack time. Sales calls can be made by these people when their time is not needed in rendering patient care.

The second issue facing home health care agencies is whether those responsible for sales should be foremost a sales professional who has learned the agency's products and services or primarily a health care professional schooled in sales techniques. In a large part, the discussion of the role of power persuaders answers the question. Health care professionals, such as nurses, can expect more ready respect from those to whom they will be selling: other health care professionals, such as discharge planners and medical doctors. Also, health care professionals enjoy a level of respect from the general public that is much higher than that of people who sell aluminum siding, for example. Finally, good professional sales techniques can be learned by anyone who has average intelligence and concern for other people's needs.

Sales training is available from a variety of sources and in a variety of formats. Colleges, sales training organizations, and consultants offer training in professional selling. Formats include classroom teaching, public and private seminars, and videotapes or audio tapes. Training styles vary with the type of selling being taught. Evaluate any program carefully to see that the style being taught matches your agency's philosophy and style.

MOTIVATING THE SALES FORCE

Motivating the sales force can pose problems for management. Too often management assumes that salespeople are motivated only by money in the form of salary, bonuses, and commissions. According to classic management theory (Herzberg, 1966), pay, along with working conditions, supervision, status, and security, does not motivate employees. Rather, achievement, recognition, responsibility, advancement, and growth motivates them. Sales awards, commendations, and the feeling of a job well done more effectively motivate salespeople than do quarterly bonuses or raises.

Salespeople are unique in the amount of rejection they must face in doing their job. Therefore, understanding, empathy, and encouragement from management is necessary to keep salespeople motivated. Some salespeople keep their motivation high by routinely listening to motivational audio tapes or attending motivational, positive thinking, seminars. To aid the efforts of the agency's management in motivating salespeople, management may find it effective to encourage the sales force to participate in such seminars or to acquire a library of motivational materials. Details of managing salespeople will be discussed in the next chapter.

CONCLUSION

Professional personal selling can be a powerful part of an agency's marketing mix. Modern consultative sales techniques help both the agency and its clients meet their mutual goals and objectives. Professional selling can be instrumental in creating and maintaining an agency's image of professionalism and quality. Selling techniques can be learned by anyone who believes in their agency and its services.

REFERENCES

Anderson, B. R. *Professional Selling* (3rd ed.). Englewood Cliffs, NJ: Prentice-Hall, 1987.

Elsea, J. G. *The Four-Minute Sales Call.* New York: Simon and Schuster, 1984.

Hanah, M. *Consultative Selling* (3rd ed.). New York: AMACOM, 1986.

Herzberg, F. *Work and the Nature of Man.* Cleveland: World Publishing, 1966.

Johnson, S., Wilson, L. *The One Minute Sales Person.* New York: William Morrow, 1984.

Kotler, P. *Marketing Management* (5th ed.). Englewood Cliffs, NJ: Prentice-Hall, 1984.

Kotler, P. *Principles of Marketing.* Englewood Cliffs, NJ: Prentice-Hall, 1980.

Legg, D., Lamb, C. W. The role of referral agents in the marketing of home health services. *Journal of Health Care Marketing.* 6(March 1986):51–56.

Manning, G. L., Reece, B. L. *Selling Today: A Personal Approach* (3rd ed.). Dubuque, IA: William C. Brown, 1987.

McDaniel, C., Darden, W. R. *Marketing.* Boston: Allyn and Bacon, 1987.

Molloy, J. T. *Dress for Success.* New York: Peter H. Wyden, 1975.

Molloy, J. T. *Live for Success.* New York: William Morrow, 1981.

Molloy, J. T. *The Woman's Dress for Success Book.* New York: Warner, 1977.

Mundinger, M. O'Niel. *Home Care Controversy: Too Little, Too Late, Too Costly.* Rockville, MD: Aspen, 1983.

Petit, T. A., McEnally, M. R., Putting strategy into promotional mix decisions. *Journal of Consumer Marketing.* 2(4)(Winter 1985):41–47.

Ponzurick, E. S., Ponzurick, T. G., Abercrombie, C. L. (1987) Marketing home health care services to the referring physician: a preliminary analysis. *Health Marketing Quarterly.* 4(3/4),47–60.

Thourlby, W. *You Are What You Wear.* New York: New American Library, 1980.

What to say in the physician's office: recognizing physician diversity. *Home Care Marketer.* 1(September 1985):3, 6.

11

Management of Time, Sales Territories, and Salespeople

The world is full of inequalities. Some people have more money, higher intelligence, better education, or better looks than others. However, one factor is the same for everyone: time. Everyone gets approximately 24 hours per day. The difference in people's accomplishments is not the time they have but, rather, how they utilize it (Mackenzie 1972). The effective use of time is important to everyone, but particularly to salespeople, home health care workers, managers, and administrators—in other words, people whose work is done without the benefit of close supervision.

TIME MANAGEMENT

The effective management of time requires two distinct processes. The first is the understanding of the limitation of demands on one's time. The second involves techniques of prioritizing activities. Every day each of us faces three types of activities: those that must be done, those that should be done, and those that we would like to do.

The only activities a human being must do are eat, sleep, and drink water. However, the reality of modern life is that, in addition to those activities, one must also work, provide shelter, and share family responsibilities. One result of the mismanagement of time is that too many activities are categoriced as "must" activities. The danger is particularly acute for women who succumb to the "superwoman" syndrome (Shaevitz, 1984). The superwoman tries to fulfill all the expectations of the roles of mother, housekeeper, working woman, and spouse. As a result, all of that person's activities are "must do," with few in the "should do" category, and none in the "would like to" list.

If you have fallen into the superwoman category, one solution (and it also works for men who cannot control their time) is to just say no (Silcox and Moore, 1980) to unwanted or unneeded activities. Surprisingly, those activities will get done adequately without your help. Saying no becomes easier after the first time. When you have clear-cut goals and priorities, saying no to those activities that do not fit your goals is easier still (Dayton, 1980). Just as having a mission focuses the business organization's efforts (see Chapter 1), having clear personal goals can help focus and prioritize one's own activities.

The second philosophy of successful time management is prioritizing one's activities. However, two schools of thought exist as to how one should prioritize. One school suggests that the best way to get things done each day is to do your most unpleasant tasks first. This way your mind will not be cluttered with thinking about an unpleasant task that must still be done. A clear mind is better able to concentrate on the remaining, more pleasant tasks.

The second method of prioritizing is at the beginning of every day to make a list of all the activities that need to be done. Assign each activity a priority as follows: (A) must be done today, (B) must be done within the next few days, (C) must be done within the next 2 weeks, and (D) must be done sometime in the future. This system centers one's attention on the most immediate tasks and provides a running tally of accomplishments by crossing completed tasks off the list. After a task is completed, one consults the list and asks, "What is the best use of my time right now?" (Lakein, 1973: 96). A modification of this approach is to prepare the list of prioritized activities at night before retiring. With all your activities planned for the next day, a good night's sleep is more probable.

The largest impediment to successful time management is procrastination: the "behavior of postponing activities." (Burka and Yuen, 1983: 5). Procrastination comes from the single source of fear: fear of success, fear of failure, desire for perfection, or distastefulness of the task, to name a few. While there are probably as many solutions to procrastination as there are authors on the subject, Burka and Yuen (1983) suggest these strategies: (1) set achievable goals and then gradually more demanding goals; (2) make a time schedule for yourself and keep track of the amount of time spent working on a particular goal; (3) enlist the support of others; and (4) deal with stress that may be reducing efficiency.

If you or your employees suffer from procrastination (even in developing a market plan) deal with the problem directly. Time management should be important to the manager or administrator of the home health care agency for both business and personal reasons. Faithful application of time management principles allows the administrator to set the standard of efficient behavior and operation expected in the organization. The efficient use of time allows the agency to be managed in a thoughtful, purposeful, and effective manner.

Without time management, administrators are drawn to less effective, less efficient management by muddling through. Muddling through is a process of dealing with situations on a unprioritized, piecemeal basis without an overall plan or purpose, which results in unintended consequences (Lindblom, 1959). An alternative—and equally unattractive—management style is management by crisis. Without priorities for activities and goals, managers deal with whatever crisis is at hand. (Typically, if the manager does not have a crisis, he or she will find one.) Again, the end results are unintended consequences and lack of attention to the true priorities of the agency.

On a personal level, the administrator who uses time management principles in his or her personal life will find more time to do the activities he or she wants to do, such as spending time with family or pursuing hobbies. A more efficient personal life allows the administrator to be more focused on business matters when at work.

Subordinates, other employees of the agency, will enjoy the same benefits when principles of time management are learned and applied. Subordinates enjoy the feeling of accomplishment in getting more done when time is managed effectively. Likewise, with more efficient private lives, employees are better able to focus on their work assignments.

An adage of management is, "People are our most important asset." This statement means that any home health care agency can buy the same equipment, but not all agencies can hire the same full-time people, and therein lies the uniqueness of the individual agency. Just as automobile engines are tuned and lubricated to obtain peak performance and efficiency, training oneself and one's employees in time management helps develop peak performance. Your agency may have the best staff and a sophisticated marketing program, and may provide the highest-quality care, but if you or your people are wasting time, you might as well be writing checks to your competition.

TERRITORY MANAGEMENT

Territory management is the concept of time management applied to the salesperson's responsibility of making contacts with established and prospective clients. If you have one full-time salesperson who covers a 50- by 50-mile area (about the area of a medium-sized city) and this person makes only two trips across the territory per day, that person is driving 44,000 miles a year. At 20.5 cents per mile. That's over $9,000 in automobile expenses. More important, even if it were possible to average 50 miles an hour driving in a metropolitan area, that person is spending over 2 full days a week doing nothing but driving a car. The primary objective of any salesperson should be spending time identifying and meeting clients' needs, not driving a car. Territory management helps influence a salesperson's activities to reduce nonproductive time, such as driving, and maximize productive time spent with clients. (Territory management can also be used to increase the efficiency of home health care nurses who make multiple visits during a day.)

Second, territory management focuses an agency's attention on important clients. (The salesperson's adage is, "All clients are important, but some are more important than others.") Vilfredo Pareto, an Italian engineer in the late nineteenth century, determined that wealth and income are not distributed equally (Twedt, 1986). Applied to marketing, Pareto's law says that if you list your clients from the largest to the smallest, the first 20% (in numbers) will account for 80% of the agency's dollar volume. Therefore, the top 20% of clients, who provide 80% of your business, should receive more attention and more frequent sales calls than the other 80%.

Third, territory management provides agency sales personnel a framework for prospecting, or looking for and developing new relationships and clients. Those who can use the services of your agency, but as yet have not, should not be ignored. The area a salesperson covers should be analyzed to determine where potential clients exist, and estimates should be made of dollar volume potential.

To design an effective territory management plan, first list clients from highest dollar volume to lowest. Next, list potential clients from highest dollar potential to lowest. (The same names can appear on both lists.) Determine the top 20% of both lists. These organizations are your A list. They should be called on most frequently. The next 50% of the names on the lists are B clients and should be called on routinely but less frequently. The remainder of this list is made up of C clients, who should be contacted whenever time allows.

The next step is to analyze the geographic distribution of these clients. Using an appropriate-sized map, put color-coded pins at each client's location. Clusters or patterns should appear. These define a territory's sectors. Now a salesperson can focus on a sector and travel to clients efficiently. Whether a salesperson's focus on a particular sector will be daily, weekly, or monthly depends on two variables: first and most important, how often the client *needs* to have contact with your organization in order to conduct business efficiently; and second, how often your competition is contacting these people. As was illustrated in Chapter 10, professional selling helps a client solve problems. Badgering clients or standing over their shoulder does not help solve their problems or produce sales for your agency. Conversely, lack of attention to any client or potential client will most certainly result in their reduction or loss of business. It is entirely possible that a client is so large that daily contact is advised.

The list of C clients, those whose volume potential is small, provides an opportunity to make efficient use of one's time. For example, if a salesperson has some extra time as a result of an appointment being canceled or a call taking less time than expected, that extra time can be used to call on the C clients. Therefore, an efficient salesperson should always have a list of C clients for each geographic sector.

A salesperson should schedule his or her time loosely enough to allow flexibility in spending time with clients. It is a no-win situation if one has to interrupt a productive but lengthy sales call to phone another client to explain that you will be late for your appointment. Appointments should be scheduled based on experience with such factors as the client's penchant for punctuality (your and theirs), the anticipated length of the sales call based on the number of objectives you want to cover, and the typical driving time between clients. Valuable time is wasted if a salesperson allows an extra 15 or 30 minutes in case there is a traffic jam or if the salesperson has a flat tire.

Conducting a territory analysis and developing a territory call plan not only identify and focus an agency's attention on the clients with the largest potential but also equalize attention among clients of similar size. In any group of clients, some are going to be more pleasant, even more fun, to deal with than others. The human tendency is to see those clients we like more frequently than those we do not. Using a call plan forces the salesperson to pay attention to clients based on dollar volume rather than personalities.

The foregoing discussion of territory analysis and call plan development used dollar volume and potential dollar volume as the basis for classifying clients. The standard an agency uses need not be dollar volume but may be referral volume (number of referrals generated). Depending on the agency's goals and target market, any measurable standard can be used as long as it reflects the agency's objectives and mission. In addition, the call plan can be modified to reflect and emphasize targeted markets. For instance, if the management of the agency has made the strategic decision to grow in the area of sick-day care for children, management can state that for client classification purposes all day care centers will be classified A for the next 6 months. The result of this action would be an intense effort by the sales force to identify the needs of and develop this targeted market.

Territory management provides analysis and guidelines useful in maximizing the efficiency of salespeople's time. It helps ensure that the limited resource time is distributed equitably and wisely among clients. Furthermore, territory management can be another tool management can use to reflect the agency's goals and target markets.

SALES FORCE MANAGEMENT

A salesperson is a unique individual. He or she must have an ego strong enough to handle frequent rejections, yet be empathetic enough to understand clients' needs. In addition, the person usually works without any direct supervision and receives no feedback from management except for reports of dollars or referrals generated. Therefore, how does the agency's management supervise and motivate those involved in sales?

First, agency management should be involved in the agency's sales effort. Making sales calls with the salesperson provides management with the following benefits: it provides first-hand information about the client's needs, helps create a stronger bond between the agency and the client, and by observation provides information about the salesperson's performance.

Clients gain more information about an agency's image, philosophy, and quality of care when the agency's management is known to them. Clients gain more confidence in an agency when they know whom they are dealing with and know whom to call to resolve a problem. Management involvement in client contacts helps build the trust between organizations needed to develop long-term relationships. In addition, management attention to clients provides a continuity in the relationship should the salesperson cease dealing with the client due to reassignment or leaving the agency.

Management calling with salespeople provides direct observation of the salesperson's efforts. Management can subjectively evaluate the person's relationship with the client. Also, management can evaluate the salesperson's judgment and analysis of the client's needs by comparing its observations with those of the salesperson. Management can also evaluate the behavior of the salesperson to see if the person's activities are in line with the policies of the agency.

Another method of managing a sales force is through compensation. However, compensating a sales force is problematical, particularly when what is being sold is health care. Commission-only compensation is the simplest (no results, no pay) and entirely results oriented. However, management has a minimum of control over the activities of commission-only salespeople. A commission-only compensation plan creates short-term results at the expense of long-term opportunities. Quick sales, the sale of unneeded services, and inhibition of the empathetic interaction needed to successfully identify and meet the client's needs all can result from commission-only sales force compensation plan (Engel et al., 1986). Therefore, commission-only compensation is unsuitable for home health care agencies.

At the other end of the compensation spectrum is salary only. Regardless of performance, the person is paid a straight salary. With this method, management has maximum control over the salesperson's activities. Results are obtained through goal-setting procedures, such as management by objectives (also known as MBO) (Drucker, 1954; Odiorne, 1965; Schleh, 1965). The behavior and traits, as well as the sales performance, of salespeople can also be evaluated through other techniques such as behaviorally anchored rating scales or BARS (Campbell, 1973). Salespeople are encouraged to perform well because of the expectation that superior performance will result in increased salaries. This system encourages long-term results but not necessarily at the expense of short-term results.

Between these two compensation plans is a range of compensation plans combining both salary and commission or bonus. If your agency adopts a consultative or partnership approach to sales, probably the most successful compensation plan will be salary-only or salary plus annual bonus for the top performers.

Management has the responsibility of determining on what criteria the performance of the sales force will be measured. Any measurable criteria can be chosen. However, the criteria must reflect the goals and mission of the agency. Criteria may include total dollar volume increase, new clients, increases in volume at existing clients, number of calls made, accuracy of reporting competitive activities, professional demeanor and appearance, participation in professional associations, success in developing new service or market opportunities, or any combination of these. Care must be taken in determining on what factors performance ratings will be based, as the sales force will rapidly adjust its activities to maximize each individual's performance. For example, if number of calls made is the criterion for performance, salespeople may sacrifice lengthy, productive calls in favor of short, nonproductive ones. Performance will look good according to the criteria set out, but the agency may not benefit from the activity.

Dollar volume increases are probably the most prevalent criteria used in evaluating sales force performance. Dollar volume increases create growth for the home health agency. However, this criterion is not without drawbacks or areas of concern for managers. For example, how should the performance of a person who historically has been a top performer be evaluated if his or her largest client, a hospital, initiates its own home care program, causing a significant drop in revenue generated? Or how should performance be evaluated if total dollars increases are the result of increased prices or reimbursement levels rather than through additional visits or clients? Such unintended outcomes should be anticipated by developing policies or contingency plans.

The number of new clients or referral sources generated can be an attractive criterion. Not only does this criterion encourage growth in agency, but it also presumes that new clients and referral sources will generate repeat business more easily. However, this criterion, too, has drawbacks. If the number of new clients or referrals sources generated is the sole basis for judging performance, salespeople may work on developing new clients while neglecting established, historical clients and sources of referrals.

Accurate and timely reporting of competitors' actions is clearly a necessary and useful function of the sales force. The professional appearance and demeanor of a salesperson, as well as a salesperson's participation in professional activities, can be a significant factor in creating the professional, quality-conscious image that management desires for the agency. However, if these are the only criteria, the result would probably be a very good looking sales force and an abundance of competitive information but declining sales dollars.

In designing the criteria by which to judge sales performance, a combination of criteria can be used. Each criterion is given a weight or factor reflecting the relative importance of that behavior or result to the agency's management. Most important, the criteria and their weighting factors must be explained to the sales force along with rules or contingency plans covering events beyond the control of management or the sales force.

CONCLUSION

The management of time, territory, and salespeople improves the efficiency and effectiveness of a home health care agency. Separately, each factor can improve an individual's performance. Collectively, they can be critical to the success of the agency.

REFERENCES

Burka, J. B., Yuen, M. *Procrastination.* Reading, MA: Addison-Wesley, 1983.

Campbell, J. P. The development and evaluation of behaviorally based rating scales. *Journal of Applied Psychology.* 58(February, 1973):15–22.

Dayton, E. R. *Tools for Time Management.* Grand Rapids, MI: Zondervan, 1980.

Drucker, P. F. *The Practice of Management.* New York: Harper & Brothers, 1954.

Engel, J. F., Blackwell, R. D., Miniard, P. W. *Consumer Behavior* (5th ed.). Chicago: Dryden Press, 1986.

Lakein, A. *How to Get Control of Your Time and Life.* New York: New American Library, 1973.

Lindblom, C. E. The science of muddling through. *Public Administration Review.* 19(1959):78–88.

Mackenzie, R. A. *The Time Trap.* New York: AMACOM, 1972.

Odiorne, G. S. *Management by Objectives.* New York: Pitman, 1965.

Schleh, E. C. *Management by Results.* New York: McGraw-Hill, 1965.

Shaevitz, M. Hansen. *The Superwoman Syndrome.* New York: Warner, 1984.

Silcox, D., Moore, M. E. *Woman Time.* New York: Wydon, 1980.

Twedt, D. W. The concept of market segmentation in *Handbook of Modern Marketing* (2nd ed.). Buell, V. P. (ed.). New York: McGraw-Hill, 1986.

PART 4

Evaluating the Role of the Home Health Care Marketer

12

Marketing Responsibility

Marketing is not undertaken simply by naming someone to the job. The term marketing still raises eyebrows in health care, and when a marketing person is introduced into the agency or named from within, care needs to be taken in orienting staff, boards, and administration as to what marketing is, how it works, and what it can do for the agency or institution.

Rubright and MacDonald (1981: 211) describe some of the considerations the administrator of an agency needs to think about when examining marketing for the agency:

1. Marketer on the organization chart
2. Orientation of all staff to marketing
3. Qualifications of a marketing person
4. Use of outside marketing consultants
5. Use of in-house marketing team
6. Building and maintaining marketing momentum

Each of these considerations will be discussed below.

ORGANIZATIONAL CHART

The administrator of the agency needs to have a close relationship with the marketing program. The marketer in turn needs access to and leverage with management. Marketing has a connection to the planning and public relations people, but it transcends all of them. Marketing comprehends all of those programs. Kotler (Mistarz, 1984: 22) notes that initially "marketing was an orphan" and that planning and public relations "did not want to claim them." Today "all are claiming this orphan called marketing," although "marketing may be the parent rather than the child of these functions." In many agencies a single person will serve in one if not all three capacities. More important is that the agency has a marketing orientation. Without a marketing orientation, it will be difficult for the marketer to accomplish marketing planning and implementation within the agency.

Kotler and Clarke (1987) suggest that, if a marketer is placed in a lower-level position, the person rarely is given the authority to do anything significant with the marketing data. The person does not have the power to implement strategies or to participate in strategy.

Often this is the type of person a home health agency hires because it can pay the person a lower salary.

In contrast, if marketing is in a vice president, director, or manager position, it shows that administration believes this person should be working closely with top management. One of the problems with this type of position is finding someone who has both the marketing and home care or health care experience.

Where the marketing person is placed on the organizational chart will depend on several factors: type of agency, full or part-time marketing position, size of agency, and level of authority.

If the home care agency is hospital based, questions arise as to whether it needs someone and whether the home care department will hire someone or a corporate or central marketing department will market all services of the institution. Figure 12.1 demonstrates an example of the central marketing concept.

Some of the smaller community-based home health agencies have staff that fill this position part-time. This makes some difference.

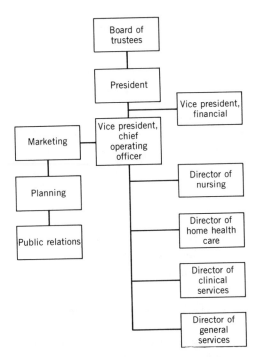

Figure 12.1. Hospital-based home care.

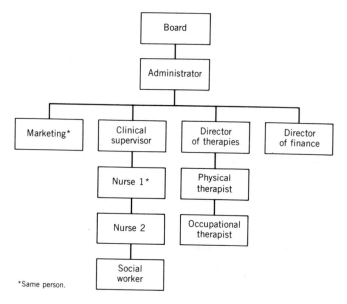

Figure 12.2. *Part-time marketing person in a home health agency.*

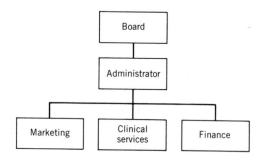

Figure 12.3. *Full-time marketing person in a home health agency.*

Often this person serves a clinical plus a marketing role. This often causes confusion on the staff's part as to whether the person is management or staff. Figure 12.2 demonstrates how this type of organization might be structured.

Figure 12.3 depicts the structure of an agency that has a full-time marketing person.

If an agency is part of a corporation, a dotted line of responsibility is added from the local marketing director to the director of marketing at the corporate level. In this instance, the marketing person is responsible not only to the agency's administrator but also to the corporate marketing manager.

Believing in marketing and explaining what it is needs to be done next with select committees and the staff. Often an agency has a planning committee or staff committee. These are the people to start with by holding sessions on what marketing is, who will do it in this agency, what their role will be, why it is being done, and the role of the staff in the overall marketing function of the agency. Continuing in-service education courses need to be given to update staff on how the plans and marketing functions are progressing.

QUALIFICATIONS OF THE MARKETER

There is currently a lot of discussion as to the qualifications of a marketing person. Do you hire someone who is doing marketing in industry, or do you hire a health care person and teach them marketing? It is probably more feasible for the home health agency to train one of its own staff about marketing because they have a sound base in health care and possess many of the planning skills needed. Whatever the agency decides, Rubright and MacDonald (1981) suggest how to increase the qualification of the person. If the person has no marketing experience the person should

1. Take marketing courses in community colleges or universities
2. Attend seminars in marketing
3. Be temporarily provided a part-time consultant, experienced in marketing
4. Acquire books and articles on marketing
5. Participate in activities of the local and national marketing association

If the agency hires someone with marketing skills but no health care experience or no home health care experience, the process is done in reverse. The person needs to be exposed to the entire workings of the agency and its profession. This is done by (Rubright and MacDonald, 1981: 216)

1. Orientation to the daily operations of each part of the agency
2. Accompanying staff on home visits

3. Participation in management meetings at all levels of the organization

4. Participation in appropriate inservice or staff development programs

The marketer should possess some general skills (Rubright and MacDonald, 1981: 216):

1. An ability to organize work well

2. An ability to command respect from all levels in the organization

3. An ability to write well

4. A sense of creativity

5. A better than ordinary degree of political sensitivity

6. An ability to converse and run meetings expeditiously

7. An ability to be objective

8. An ability to mediate differences between groups

Weinrauch (1987: 15) also suggests characteristics of a successful marketer. Such a person

1. Is innovative and entrepreneurial in thought and actions

2. Appreciates the financial dimensions of marketing actions

3. Knows how to promote products and services

4. Is mentally agile, dependable, and technically competent

5. Appreciates the multitude of factors that affect pricing discussions

6. Is able to monitor and predict necessary channel changes

7. Knows how to plan and implement the strategic and tactical elements of a marketing program

8. Can predict future trends in sales, cost, and client interest

9. Looks constantly for ways to improve the marketing intelligence within the organization

These characteristics stress the entrepreneurial and financial role of the marketer. Whoever the person is, good people skills, planning, market research, objectivity, and financial knowledge are skills the person should possess.

OUTSIDE CONSULTANT

If an outside consultant is used, the consultant should possess all the qualifications previously mentioned. The value of the outside consultant depends largely on the quality of outside expertise. Because health care marketing is so new, many marketing firms do not have this expertise. Consultants can be used a variety of ways. One would be to have a consultant provide market training for staff and volunteers. This would help staff to better understand what marketing is and what their role will be. Another way is to hire the consultant on a retainer basis to offer regular consultation to the marketer. For example, the agency could formulate a market plan and use the consultant to help analyze the results and define strategies to address identified problems. Still another way is to contract with a consultant to do a specific project that the market department does not have the skills, time, or equipment to do. This is often in the area of market research when the agency needs objective data on which to base a decision.

Outside help can benefit the organization greatly, but there are also problems. Kotler and Clark (1987: 141) state "that health care organizations that rely on outside expertise face one of two problems":

1. The outside expert addresses not only a series of small marketing issues but also major strategic marketing issues that affect the agency over the long term. The problem is the cost of such an effort, provided by an outside consultant, can be astronomical.

2. If outside expertise is brought in to address only the small marketing problems, no one is addressing the larger issues that have long-term implications. This piecemeal approach could leave the organization with an inconsistent or no marketing strategy.

Hiring a Consultant

If a consultant is to be used, the agency needs to spend time to locate a consultant who matches the agency. Steps in hiring a consultant are as follows:

1. Determine what the agency wants the consultant to do.
2. Gather information on consultants or firms.

3. Select the consultant or firm.

4. Write the agreement.

5. Proceed with the designated task.

Step 1 is very important. If the agency cannot specifically state what it needs or wants, it is difficult for the consultant to know what is expected, and the agency may not receive the end product it expected.

If the agency spends time defining the areas where it needs assistance, the consultant knows how to address the agency's needs. The agency should also decide how much it is going to spend and set that as a ceiling.

Step 2 entails gathering information on consultants or firms. When selecting who to work with, the agency needs to explore various people and firms. To find a good consultant, contact the local chapter of the American Marketing Association, local universities, national marketing associations, speakers at marketing seminars, authors of marketing books, or—the best source—other agencies or individuals who have used various consultants.

Step 3 involves selecting the consultant that best matches the agency. The agency should interview the prospective consultant or individuals from the firm. References should be requested if you do not know the person. If a large project is to be done, some agencies request a proposal from the consultant. This enables the agency to know in detail how a consultant would complete the designated task. It also shows how the consultant would cost out the project. Each proposal should be carefully reviewed, and the one that meets the agencies needs accepted.

Once the firm or consultant has been selected, a letter of agreement or a formal contract should be written, depending on the circumstances. Many agencies are reluctant to sign agreements, but such agreements protect both the agency and the consultant so they will not have to rely on their memory. The agreement should state the following:

1. When the project should start and end

2. What the consultant will provide and what the agency will provide

3. What final product is expected

4. Cost agreed upon

Holtz (1983: 241) suggests that the agreement "specify anything and everything that represents items of cost, items for which you make specific charges, and/or items which represent to the client what he or she is buying." The amount of detail in an agreement ultimately depends on what the agency and the consultant feel comfortable with.

IN-HOUSE MARKETING

Because successful marketing depends on the commitment and enthusiasm of the staff, in-house marketing is best. In-house marketing can be done by the marketer or a marketing committee, depending on the wishes of the agency.

Criteria for selecting people to serve on a marketing team include

1. Belief in and familiarity with marketing
2. Knowledge of the specific marketing subject or project
3. Knowledge of the potential target group
4. Interest in the project
5. Good interpersonal skills
6. Creative thinking
7. Planning skills

A representation from across the staff will produce the most well-balanced team. Each different department or level will add input that will prevent special interests from being overpromoted.

Marketing teams should be kept small to facilitate the group process. Membership can run from four to ten people for a workable team. Once a team leader has been specified, the leader should

1. Convene the marketing team and discuss charges, the project, and dates for meetings.
2. Agree on the approach to the project.
3. Define objectives of the project.
4. Identify key dates for project.
5. Identify opportunities and threats to the project.
6. Conduct research studies about the project.

7. Identify and review the target audience.

8. Define suggested strategies.

9. Analyze resources and evaluate strategies.

10. Prepare a market plan for that strategy.

11. Submit the recommended strategy to management for approval.

12. Once approval is received, implement the strategy according to the market plan.

13. Evaluate the results of the strategy.

14. Modify the strategy as needed.

Often it is hard in home care to get everyone together for meetings because members of the team are not always at the agency. Assigning duties and then holding periodic meetings to coordinate all activities is one way that such problems can be overcome.

If time and money are spent educating staff members on how to develop market plans, audits, and evaluation, the agency will get a long-term return on their money.

MOMENTUM

Momentum depends on commitment. Many agencies hire a marketing director or give someone a marketing title to demonstrate that they have a marketing orientation. Many agencies are not sure what to do with this person once hired, but because everyone else has a marketing manager they feel they should too. Commitment from the administration needs to be visible to the marketing people and to all staff members. Support, which includes funding, resources, and authority, needs to be continued on a long-term basis, not just at the start.

The marketing manager can maintain the momentum by keeping staff members informed and by asking for their input and feedback on implemented strategies and new ideas.

It is also important that mechanisms are set up to allow the staff to have input. The marketing manager should attend some of the weekly team meetings, orientation sessions, or whatever staff meetings the agency has. This makes the person more visible and suggests that he or she wants feedback.

The other essential component is that once staff members or managers give input, they need to hear what was done about their idea or input. Writing a note to such people shows them that their input is valued and acknowledged and lets them know what is being done. No one likes to give suggestions and then see the program or service go on exactly as before with no word of what happened to their suggestion. People soon stop giving feedback.

The momentum will stay with staff members if they feel a sense of pride and accomplishment in the work the agency has done to better meet the needs of the clients. However, staff members sometimes need more than just a feeling of pride. Incentives for doing a good marketing job should be given. Incentives can be anything from a letter of recognition in a personnel file to cash. Recognition dinners are one method some agencies use to recognize outstanding staff members. Other incentives include plaques, employee-of-the-month awards, or an upgrading of an employee's job title.

Cash incentives work in various ways. Some agencies set goals of a certain number of referrals per month and pay a bonus for referrals in excess of that number. Other agencies pay staff extra for those visits made after the expected number per day. Agencies may also offer staff members and managers greater participation in profit sharing in the agency.

All incentives help to motivate the staff, but an agency needs to determine what incentives are appropriate for its staff. Whether the incentive is secure employment, recognition, or cash, it must closely match with the philosophy of the agency.

CONCLUSION

Marketing is not undertaken simply by naming someone to the job. It involves orienting administration and staff to what marketing is and how all personnel will be involved.

Where the marketing manager is placed in the agency varies with the size of the agency, the type of agency, and whether the job is a full- or part-time position. The main point is that the marketing person needs access to management and needs some authority to carry out marketing functions for the agency.

Certain attributes are highly desirable in a marketing person. The organization should consider whether it will use an in-house marketing person or an outside consultant. Using a blend of in-house marketing and outside consulting is often the best.

The marketing manager is not solely responsible for marketing;

rather, marketing should take a team approach. Staff members should be included in marketing planning and strategy development. Maintaining the marketing momentum for staff and management is a challenge that must be accepted, and rewards should be given for doing a good marketing job.

REFERENCES

Cebrzynski, G. Marketing, tradition clash in health care. *Marketing News.* 19(November 1985):1, 30.

Holtz, H. *How to Succeed as an Independent Consultant.* New York: John Wiley & Sons, 1983.

Kotler, P., Clarke, R. *Marketing for Health Care Organizations.* Englewood Cliffs, NJ: Prentice-Hall, 1987.

Mistarz, J. The evolution of marketing in hospitals. *Hospitals Factbook.* (1984):22.

Rubright, R., MacDonald, D. *Marketing Health and Human Services.* Rockville, MD: Aspen, 1981.

Weinrauch, J. *The Marketing Problem Solver.* New York: John Wiley & Sons, 1986.

13

Marketing
Ethics

Chapter 1 discussed why marketing health care is ethical, but what are the ethics of marketing? Marketing ethics are a subset of the larger concept of business ethics. In addition, business ethics are related to but separate from the concept of the social responsibility of a business. Social responsibility generally encompasses a "set of generally accepted relationships, obligations, and duties between institutions and the people" (Steiner, 1972). Some people believe that because corporations exist at the pleasure of society, corporations therefore have a responsibility to society as a whole. The economist Milton Friedman (1970) believes that the only socially responsible action a business can take is to make as large a profit as is possible acting within the law.

Ethics deal with questions of right and wrong. The medical profession has been more successful than the business community in establishing ethical standards of behavior (Machan and Den Uyl, 1987). Finding one set of guidelines that fits all situations is the challenge—as yet unmet—of those studying marketing ethics.

The following example illustrates one dilemma in trying to judge whether a business or marketing decision is ethical. The Medicaid benefits of a client of a home health care agency have expired. The home health nurse, along with his or her supervisors, agree that, based on medical reasons alone, the care should be continued. However, for some reason the referring physician has been unable or unwilling to sign orders for continued care. The supervisors know that if records are falsified a certain way, reimbursement for continued care is certain. What is the ethical response to this situation?

This example illustrates the two basic types of assumptions regarding ethical behavior. Should the action be judged as ethical or unethical, or should the results of the action be judged as ethical or unethical? Philosophers refer to consideration of the "inherent righteous of a behavior" (Hunt and Vitell, 1986: 6) as deontological, whereas "teleological philosophies deal with the moral worth of a behavior determined totally by the consequences of the behavior" (Ferrell and Gresham, 1985: 89). More simply put, do the ends justify the means (teleological), or does the means justify the ends (deontological)?

Whether one takes a deontological or teleological view of ethics will determine what one considers the ethical action in the foregoing example. A deontological view would be that violating the law and lying are inherently wrong (unethical); therefore, documents will not be falsified, and care will either be stopped or continued without reimbursement. Conversely, a teleological view would be that the inherent good in continuing needed care outweighs any perceived wrong in lying or violating the law. Under each of these views are a number of ethical philosophies that provide guidelines for judging behavior. Several of these philosophies will be discussed here.

PHILOSOPHIES OF ETHICS

One deontological view is that ethical behavior is, or should be, embodied in the law. "If it's legal, it's ethical" is the guideline. Ruth Roemer (1987), of the American Public Health Association, appears to support this view and implies that action should be taken to influence the making of laws that can form an ethical basis for action.

Immanuel Kant (Kant, 1964; originally published 1785) created much of the reasoning for deontology, based on two concepts. First, the "only possible basis for establishing a moral tradition is human reason or logic" (Robin and Reidenbach, 1987, 46). Second, Kant proposed the "categorical imperative," meaning that the guide for action should be that "one ought never act unless one is willing to have the maxim on which one acts become a universal law" (Robin and Reidenbach, 1987, 46). The categorical imperative is somewhat of an extension of the Biblical Golden Rule: "Do unto others as you would have them do unto you." However, using the categorical imperative, whatever you do unto others, others would be required or at least allowed under law to do unto you.

A teleological view is that of utilitarianism. Utilitarianism is summarized as the greatest good for the greatest number, which is determined through cost-benefit analysis. However, the analysis must go beyond economic costs and benefits to include utility, which is generally unquantifiable (Robin and Reidenbach, 1987). Utilitarianism has been popular with business because it correlates economic efficiency with ethical behavior. Likewise, "it is unethical to engage in an act which leads to personal gain at the expense of society in general" (Ferrell and Gresham, 1985: 89). However, utilitarianism is the ethical philosophy used by Ford Motor Company to support not redesigning the Pinto's fuel system, with the result of several deaths and injuries to people involved in accidents (Dowie, 1977), and by Nestlé to initially continue selling infant formula in third world countries where the product was misused, causing the death and malnutrition of many babies (Miller, 1983). Under utilitarianism, each of these decisions was completely ethical.

Laczniak and Murphy (1985) dismiss the categorical imperative, utilitarianism, and the Golden Rule as being too simplistic to effectively guide businesspeople in marketing decisions. Laczniak (1985) proposes a series of questions that encompasses both teleological and deontological views. The presumption is that if an act can pass all eight tests, the act is probably ethical.

The questions posed by Laczniak (1985) are as follows:

1. Will the action violate any law?
2. Will the action violate any of the moral obligations?
   a. Fidelity (the duty to remain faithful to previous actions, such as upholding contracts, keeping promises, or redressing wrongful acts)
   b. Gratitude (the duty to uphold special obligations between friends and partners)
   c. Justice (the duty to distribute rewards based on merit: going beyond the letter of the law
   d. Beneficence (the obligation to do good by increasing intelligence, virtue, or the happiness of others)
   e. Self-improvement (the duty to provide one's own self-interest, particularly one's personal virtue, intelligence, and happiness)
   f. Nonmaleficence (the duty to not to injure others)
3. Does this action violate any special obligations which are the result of the type of business the organization is in? For the home health care agency, this means, Does the action violate the special obligations of any health care organization to preserve life, improve the quality of life, alleviate suffering, and provide high-quality care?
4. Is the intent of this action evil?
5. Will this action result in or cause any major evils?
6. Does an alternative to this action exist that if chosen would provide equal or more good while creating less evil?
7. Will this action infringe on any of the rights of the consumer, such as the right to safe and effective products and services?
8. Will this action leave another person, group, or organization less well off?

Laczniak (1985: 23) advises that these "questions need not be pursued in any lockstep fashion but can be discussed in an order dictated by the situation."

CREATING ETHICAL BEHAVIOR

The ethical behavior of a home health care agency is first the responsibility of each individual employee but ultimately the responsibility of the agency's management or administrators. Discussing and understanding the philosophies that judge ethical behavior is fine, but what can a manager do to create ethical marketing behavior in his or her own agency? The role that an agency's management has in creating an ethical environment cannot be overemphasized.

First, members of management should subscribe to an appropriate professional code of ethics. The National League for Nursing (NLN), the National Association of Home Care (NAHC), and the American Marketing Association (AMA) are but a few of the professional, industry, and trade groups that publish codes of ethics. As a manager, subscribe to a code of ethics, communicate that fact to your employees, and encourage or require them to subscribe to the code as well.

Second, create your agency's own code of ethics. An effective code of ethics should be specific and unambiguous, and should include provisions for enforcement and specific actions that will be taken when violations are found (Laczniak and Murphy, 1985). Such codes can be created by asking employees to identify areas of ethical concern in open and frank discussions (Dubinsky, 1985). Chonko and Hunt (1985) identified honesty as the most difficult ethical issue for marketing managers in service-oriented firms. Other ethical issues identified as of concern to marketers included bribery, fairness, and pricing.

A third step toward ethical marketing behavior is to hire ethical people (Loucks, 1987). Naturally, one cannot expect an unethical person to give an honest answer to the question, "Are you an ethical person?" However, other interviewing techniques can be more successful. Asking a job candidate to provide a solution to an ethical dilemma such as the one given earlier may elicit a "right" answer. However, an honest answer would be no different from the exaggeration expected from anyone seeking a job. A more indirect method would be to ask the interviewee to describe one of his or her notable marketing or sales successes. The marketing or sales methods the person describes can give some insight into the ethical standards under which that person operates.

Fourth, do not let yourself or your personnel become isolated (Loucks, 1987). The opportunity for unethical behavior is a prime predictor of unethical behavior (Ferrell and Gresham, 1985). Managers and administrators should encourage continuing open and frank discussions with employees. In addition, making sales calls with salespeople reduces this isolation and provides the manager with the opportunity to demonstrate desirable ethical behavior.

Fifth, managers, through their actions, must set an impeccable example of the ethical behavior expected of employees (Loucks, 1987). Managers' behavior is the "single best predictor of perceptions of the extent of ethical problems" (Chonko and Hunt, 1985: 353). The adage "actions speak louder than words" applies directly to managers creating an ethical marketing environment. More important, if the perception of unethical behavior exists inside one's organization, then the same perception will exist outside the organization, where it will adversely effect the image of the agency. Carroll (1987: 13) similarly suggests that managers must have "clear principles, a process for weighting ethical factors, and the ability to identify what are likely to be the moral, as well as economic, outcomes of a decision."

Ethics are part of corporate culture. Corporate culture is created by the actions of owners and senior management. Vernon R. Loucks, Jr. (1987, 6), chief executive officer of Baxter Travenol Laboratories, Inc., provides four principles of ethical management: "First, hire the right people; second, set standards more than rules; third, don't let yourself get isolated; fourth and most important, let your ethical example at all times be absolutely impeccable."

In any population of individuals or organizations, ethical marketing behavior will range from ethical to unethical. No business, profession, or group is immune from the presence of bad apples spoiling the bunch. Therefore, it is a virtual certainty that as home health care grows and marketing is increasingly utilized, abuses or unethical behavior will occur. When abuse occurs, does this mean that marketing was at fault? No. Sound marketing principles are not unethical. Misapplication of marketing principles by unethical people results in unethical actions.

For example, consider the case of a salesperson ambitious to earn a performance bonus who convinces an infirm person to use home care. The client's medical condition is such that hospitalization is warranted. As a result, the client dies, and the situation is reported by local news media. Who is to blame for this situation? Does the blame lie with the salesperson for attempting to earn a performance bonus? Is the salesperson's manager to blame for setting ambitious sales goals? Is the client to blame for not recognizing the seriousness of his or her medical condition? Is this situation an indictment of the home care industry? Is marketing to blame?

Only the individual can control the ethics of his or her own behavior. However, the owner, manager, or administrator has the responsibility for setting the ethical agenda for the agency and its marketing program. Employees have the choice of conforming to the ethical standards set by the agency's management or seeking employment elsewhere.

CONCLUSION

Is providing health care ethical? Is adapting one's organization to meet the needs of clients ethical? Is informing the uninformed about the availability of health care ethical? Is obtaining feedback to see if your service met the client's expectations ethical? If the answer to each of these questions is yes, then marketing home health care is ethical. However, whether an agency markets ethically can be determined only by the agency's leaders.

REFERENCES

Carroll, B. In search of a moral manager. *Business Horizons.* 30(March–April 1987):7–15.

Chonko, L. B., Hunt, S. D. Ethics and marketing management: an empirical examination. *Journal of Business Research.* 13(1985):339–359.

Dowie, M. How Ford put two million firetraps on wheels. *Business and Society Review.* (Fall 1977):46–55.

Dubinsky, A. J. Studying field salespeople's ethical problems: an approach for designing company policies in *Marketing Ethics: Guidelines for Managers.* Laczniak, G. R., Murphy, P. E. (eds.). Lexington, MA: Lexington Books, 1985.

Ferrell, D. C., Gresham, L. G. A contingency framework for understanding ethical decision making in marketing. *Journal of Marketing.* 49(Summer 1985):87–96.

Friedman, M. The social responsibility of business is to increase profits. *New York Times Magazine.* (September 13, 1970):33.

Hunt, D., Vitell, S. A general theory of marketing ethics. *Journal of Macromarketing.* 6(Spring 1986):5–15.

Kant, I. *Groundwork of the Metaphysics of Morals.* Patton, H. J. (trans.). New York: Harper & Row, 1964.

Laczniak, G. R. Framework for analyzing marketing ethics in *Marketing*

Ethics: Guidelines for Managers. Laczniak, G. R., Murphy, P. (eds.). Lexington, MA: Lexington Books, 1985.

Laczniak, G. R., Murphy, P. E. (eds.). *Marketing Ethics: Guidelines for Managers.* Lexington, MA: Lexington Books, 1985.

Loucks, V. R., Jr. A CEO looks at ethics. *Business Horizons.* 30(March–April 1987):2-6.

Machan, T. R., Den Uyl, D. J. Recent work in business ethics: a survey and critique. *American Philosophy Quarterly.* 24(April 1987):107-124.

Miller, F. D. *Out of the Mouths of Babes: The Infant Formula Controversy.* Bowling Green, OH: Social Philosophy and Policy Center, 1983.

Robin, D. R., Reidenbach, R. Social responsibility, ethics, and marketing strategy: closing the gap between concept and application. *Journal of Marketing.* 51(January 1987):44-58.

Roemer, R. Public health ethics and the law. *The Nation's Health.* 17(May–June 1987):2.

Steiner, G. A. Social policies for business. *California Management Review.* 14(Winter 1972):17-24.

14

Future Trends in Home Health Care

"The future of home care is very bright," says Elsie Griffith, executive officer of the Visiting Nurse Service of New York (Griffith, 1985). More recently, Griffith (1987) has identified some of the challenges home health care faces, such as combating an image of low-cost care and increasing the value put on care in the home. If the future is to be as bright as it could be, these factors will have to change.

Predicting the future is always a challenge. Futurists, such as Marvin Cetron (1985), attempt to evaluate the future quantitatively. Three factors must be taken in consideration when evaluating the future quantitatively. First is an event's probability of happening. Second is the impact a particular event has when it occurs. Multiplying these two factors together produces the third factor, which is effectiveness. For instance, if a catastrophic earthquake occurs along the San Andreas Fault and much of California slides into the ocean, the impact of that event would be very great. However, the probability of that event's happening within a person's lifetime is extremely small. Therefore, the effectiveness of that event is relatively small.

A second method used by futurists, such as John Naisbett, is content analysis (Naisbett, 1982). The Naisbett group analyzes newspapers to determine what people are concerned about and in what direction their thinking is moving, thereby establishing a trend toward the future.

A third method, used in predicting stock market prices, is called the random walk theory (McCormack, 1984). While considered a serious theory, its tenet is simple. The random walk theory holds that since the future is unforeseen, the best prediction of the future is what is known, that is, the situation as it is today. In other words, the best prediction of tomorrow's weather is today's weather. (Try it and see how often the random walk theory is accurate in predicting the weather.)

The biggest risk in attempting to predict the future lies in the assumptions that must be made. One common assumption is that current trends (straight lines) will continue. This type of assumption has lead to some notably erroneous conclusions. For example, in about 1890, based on the then current trends, it was predicted that by 1930 one third of the population of New York City would have to be employed as street sweepers to control the horse excrement!

The second risk is predicting whether an event of significant impact will occur. Quantitatively, probabilities can be calculated, but in reality, either an event will or will not occur. For example, the probability that one's death will occur as a result of a motor vehicle accident is .00024. For practical purposes, that datum is meaningless because, while one's death is certain to occur, it either will or will not be as a result of a motor vehicle accident.

When Griffith (1985) states that the future of home care is bright, she means that opportunities exist or will be created for home health care to grow and expand. The growth and expansion of home health care will be effected by five categories of changes: environmental, political, economic, technological, and demographic (social) (Cole, 1986). How each of the categories affects home health care and the assumptions made about each will be discussed here.

OVERALL ASSUMPTIONS

First, two assumptions must be made in order to assure that there is a future to predict. One is that in the foreseeable future no nuclear holocaust will occur. The second is that no worldwide conventional war will take place.

ENVIRONMENTAL CHANGES

Of all five categories of change, environmental has the smallest impact on home health care. The assumption is that within the next generation no significant changes or deterioration of the world's environment will occur. Thus, the environment will have no impact on home health care. However, this assumption may be wrong. For instance, if the greenhouse effect (the reduction of ozone in the earth's atmosphere) continues and results in the expected increase in skin cancers, a significant increase in the demand for home health care could be predicted.

POLITICAL CHANGES

The major assumption for the impact on home health care in the political category is that the United States will remain under a democratic political system. Certainly, funding for all forms of health care will be influenced by the political party in the White House. (It has been said that the difference between Republicans and Democrats is whether one sees government as the problem or the solution, respectively.)

When the federal administration changes from Republican to Democrat, the effect of this change on funding for health care is a matter of conjecture. Cetron, however, has predicted a Democrat administration will return to power in 1988 (Cetron and O'Toole, 1982). Regardless of whether this prediction is correct for the 1988 presidential elections, it is a certainty that at some time the nation's administration will change from Republican to Democrat.

Also of significant impact in the political category is the role nurses and other health professionals will play in political activism. The concern over the rising costs of health care will eventually result in the passage of legislation allowing direct reimbursement of nurses. Political activism by nurses might speed this certainty.

Also, public policy makers have yet to deal with the issues of a national health insurance program. Approval of a national health insurance or catastrophic health insurance plan will increase the demand for health care. Approval may also require the use of alternative delivery systems as a method of reducing costs. Three factors indicate that passage of some type of national health insurance plan is likely by the year 2000. First, as more people become underinsured or uninsured, public concern and awareness of the problem will grow until it becomes politically astute to support the concept. Second, as Social Security and its funds, Medicaid and Medicare, grow increasingly financially weak, public pressure will mount to find a solution. Third, medical doctors and insurance companies will join forces to support the legislation. Insurance companies will be attracted by a market mandated by law. Medical doctors faced with declining incomes will support legislation, recognizing that the resultant increased demand for their services will allow their incomes to rise.

The movement toward some form of national insurance will affect home health care. The home care industry will need to take an active role in influencing the policy decisions. Professional organizations such as the National Association of Home Care will increase their legislative activities through the involvement of their membership and through health coalitions that are forming among professional groups on issues common to all.

ECONOMIC CHANGES

Since this book focuses on home health care in the United States, a basic assumption about the future is that the United States will remain under a basically free-market, capitalistic system. Also assumed is that no catastrophic collapse of the nation's money system will occur. However, recessionary times are certain to occur, probably by 1990. Higher unemployment and the protection of fewer people by health insurance may result in a reduction of the utilization of health care facilities. An accompanying reduction in employment of nurses, in spite of a predicted shortage of registered nurses, could have two results that affect home health care. First, unemployed nurses with an entrepreneurial streak may start additional home health agencies. Second, some of these nurses may start a black market in health care, providing primary care to uninsured or underinsured persons in exchange for cash or barter.

Home health care can benefit in times of economic recession or in times of growth. Recessionary times force businesses, including hospitals, to look for more efficient ways of delivering their products or services. A desire for increased efficiency on the part of hospitals, whether or not the result of a recession, may focus attention on home health care as a more efficient method of delivering patient care. However, if economic times remain good, increased income and discretionary income are the expected results. With increased income, consumers increase their focus on the quality of life rather than on the efficiency of life or on simple economic survival. Increased attention to the quality of life gives home health care an opportunity to provide care that increases, and not just maintains, the patient's quality of life. With more discretionary income and a heightened concern for the quality of life, adult children may be more willing to provide home health care to their parents as an alternative to having the parents live in the child's home or putting the parents in a nursing home.

TECHNOLOGICAL CHANGES

Technological advances will constitute one of the greatest positive effects on home health care in the future. Naisbitt (1982) has predicted that we are moving toward a high-tech, high-touch society in which people will demand the best available technology employed in a user-friendly fashion. Increased miniaturization and improved communication will allow more sophisticated equipment and procedures to be moved into the home. Home health care is perfectly situated to take advantage of the high-tech, high-touch trend. Home health care nurses have or are developing the skills necessary to operate high-tech equipment in the home. In addition, home health care nurses are uniquely trained in assessment of the whole person, providing the high-touch factor.

DEMOGRAPHIC CHANGES

Demographic and/or social changes are the most predictable. Likewise, such changes are the most certain harbingers of future growth for home health care.

The population of the United States is aging. The baby boomers of the 1940s, 1950s, and 1960s are growing older. In addition, they are not reproducing at either a replacement rate or a growth rate. These two facts have a significant impact on the growth of home health care.

First, traditional users of home health care are the elderly. Therefore, as the population of elderly baby boomers increases, the number using home health care will certainly increase. Second, the baby boomers have taken an unprecedented interest in health and fitness. If that interest translates into increased longevity, a larger population will be available for an expanded market of home health care.

A second consideration regarding the role of the aging baby boomers is that they are creating smaller families. Therefore, fewer adult children will be available to care for their aging parents. Also, the cost of parental care will be concentrated among fewer children, increasing the financial burden and the incentive to find economical and efficient health care.

Third, the baby boomer generation has made the quality of life a priority. Therefore, it is reasonable to assume that such an emphasis will continue into their later years. Home health care has already been proven to have a significant, positive impact on the quality of life; therefore, it will be attractive to the elderly baby boomer. In addition, the baby boomers have been accused of being narcissistic—they have been called the "me" generation—and should be expected to be less tractable and less attracted to the regimen found in institutions such as nursing homes.

The trend toward two-income families and the increasing number of single-parent households also provide growth opportunities for home health care agencies. Both situations have a common factor: parents who are less able, because of work responsibilities, to care for sick children or parents. Home health care through sick day care or adult day care will expand to meet those growing needs.

There are no negative factors for the growth of home care in the future. Only regulation and legislation may alter the speed and direction of home health care growth. Future-oriented home health care personnel can affect the legislative process, creating an environment where clients can have a choice in the type of health care they receive.

A FUTURE OVERVIEW

In the not too distant future, three types of home health care agencies will exist: corporate, market oriented, and traditional. Each will serve different publics and have different philosophies guiding their existence.

Our prediction states that soon the majority of home health care agencies will be owned by big business, primarily insurance companies, hospitals, and large national home care companies. The purpose of those home health care agencies will be to serve the needs of the corporate owner by providing profits to the corporate coffers and lowering the costs of the health care provided. Insurance companies and hospitals are not known for their innovation; therefore, little opportunity will probably exist for new markets and services to be developed. It should be noted that the history of business shows that whenever a market is dominated by big business, numerous opportunities exist for entrepreneurs to fill market niches overlooked or ignored by the larger businesses.

Another variety of corporate home health care agency will develop. The home care conglomerate will center on services rendered and sold in the home. Avon is well along this course. Starting by selling only women's cosmetics door to door, Avon now sells cosmetics and toiletries for both men and women, costume jewelry, clothes, and gifts, and is now experimenting with real estate and home mortgages. Also, Avon owns Foster Medical Corporation, a durable medical equipment company. To position itself as a "total personal consultant," all Avon needs to do is to add lawn and pest control services, milk delivery, and home health care. The final step in the process will be to have the Avon representative selling *all* these products and services.

The second type of future home health care agency is market

oriented. These are the agencies who constantly listen to their clients and watch the marketplace to identify clients' needs. They will creatively attack problems presented and grow into the future. Above, an example was given of how corporate entities outside the health industry will grow into home health care. One type of market-oriented home health care agency will do the same: expand into offering all types of personal home care, including cosmetics, lawn care, life insurance, home repair, and any other product or service used or purchased in the home. Other market opportunities that these agencies can pursue are so numerous that they will be dealt with separately in the next section.

The last type of home health care agency is the traditional agency. The focus of these agencies will continue to be the securing of government or third-party payments. Services offered will change only as funding requirements change. The future success of these agencies will depend solely on their ability to stay on the right side of the fence politically.

NEW HOME HEALTH CARE MARKET OPPORTUNITIES

Opportunities abound for market-oriented home health care agencies. Pursuing these opportunities can provide society an improved quality of life, better health, and increased efficiency. The agency that successfully adapts these ideas will be providing increased job security for its employees, creating more job opportunities through expansion of their services, and generating increased income and profits.

Looking into the future requires an open mind. Therefore, as each opportunity is discussed, evaluate it critically, but with an open mind. Some of the ideas are better than others. However, if only one idea is successfully implemented by your agency but it secures your future and that of your agency's employees, wasn't the exercise worthwhile?

Direct Contracts

Home health care agencies can contract directly with labor unions, corporations, and insurance companies. A contractual agreement with a labor union could be in the form of a benefit to retired workers, a benefit to active workers, or an addendum to current health care insurance. Corporations could be contracted directly to provide home health care as a health care benefit, as a benefit to active employees with sick day care, or as a preferred provider offering employees group rates on care provided to elderly parents. It has been predicted that insurance companies will hold significant ownership in home health care agencies in the future. By establishing a relationship with an insurance company, a home health care agency could gain a population of cases provided by the insurance company. Depending on the goals of the home health care agency's owners, such a relationship could either thwart the insurance company's entry into home health care or establish a relationship that will result in the eventual profitable sale of the home health agency to the insurance company.

Sick Day Care

Working parents face a painful dilemma when a child is ill. The parent has the limited options of either taking off work or imposing on a non-working friend or relative to care for the ill child. The number of two-income families is increasing, as is the number of single-parent households. Therefore, the number of people facing this dilemma is increasing. Taking days off to care for a sick child reduces the parent's quality of life by using up vacation time or personal sick days, may result in a reduction of income due to docked wages, and may adversely influence the parent's career opportunities through a record of high absenteeism.

Sick day care, the use of a home health care agency to care for an ill child, could relieve the parent of the dilemma, protect the parent's income and career opportunities, and provide the parent with the peace of mind of knowing that the child is receiving professional health care. Sick day care could be marketed directly to parents, as benefit provided by the employer, or through an arrangement with day care centers to care for the child when ill.

Adult Day Care

As couples age, one member often becomes a care giver as the result of an illness of the other. Adult day care can provide the healthy member of a couple with a day off or with the hours from 8:00 A.M. to 5:00 P.M. every day off from the responsibilities of care giving. Likewise, if the care giver is an adult child, adult day care can provide the same services. The need for adult day care will increase because of the increasing emphasis among the elderly on the quality of life and because of the reduction in family size. In other words, in the near future, care of a parent will increasingly fall to one or two children as opposed to being shared among three to five children.

Small Retirement Homes

One predictor of the future can be the past. In the past, retirement homes were small, intimate, homelike settings with fewer than 10 residents. Home health care agencies have the skills needed to operate such a facility. The facility could either be owned by the agency (and also provide administrative offices for the agency's other services) or be operated by an agency for another owner. Aside from the advantages to the residents of being in a homelike setting, the quality of care should be higher because of the better observation of residents by observant home health care professionals.

Case Management

Every year over a million people spend the winter south of where they have lived their lives. "Snowbirds" leave behind friends, family, and relationships with health care professionals. Who looks after their health during their time in Arizona, Florida, or Texas? If your parents—whom you are accustomed to seeing weekly—are snowbirds, would you like to have the peace of mind that their health remains sound while they are wintering elsewhere? Home health care agencies in the sunbelt could contract with adult children or parents themselves to provide monthly physical assessments to monitor any changes in the parents' health and provide an early warning of any changes that should receive attention. This service could also be offered to children whose ailing parents live year round in another part of the country. The home care agency could be contracted to manage the parent's health.

Increased Communicable Disease

All home health care agencies, particularly traditional agencies, will benefit from an unfortunate expected rise in communicable diseases. Parents are immunizing their children less, with the inevitable result of increasing communicable disease rates. Tuberculosis and AIDS continue to be public health problems in today's world. This trend will result in increased demand for public health and home health care services.

MARKETING HOME HEALTH CARE AND THE FUTURE

The future of home health care is bright, but it is also filled with problems and opportunities. The future is brightest for the home health care agencies who learn the skills of marketing and apply them constantly to their efforts. The skills of marketing are applicable to any type of agency, whether corporate, market-oriented, or traditional. Marketing skills can help the traditional agency be more effective in securing funding and managing community relations. Marketing skills can help both the corporate and market-oriented agency adapt to meet the consumers' needs.

However, much must be done if home health care is to achieve its full potential of improving clients' health and quality of life. First, home health care agencies must learn to promote and market themselves and their services. Cetron's study (1985) vividly showed that a large majority (61%) of surveyed individuals are not aware that home health care exists. However, of those who are aware of home health care services, 85% have a positive attitude toward home health care. Thus, home health care is one of the nation's best-kept secrets. Therefore, the first step home health care agencies must take into the future must be to increase awareness of their existence and the benefits they can provide.

Second, additional market research must be done to identify and quantify the needs that can be met through home health care. The ideas suggested here are the results of creative thinking and the extension of existing data. Whether they can be reinforced with empirical data or translated into successes for home health care agencies remains to be seen.

Third, home health care agencies must be involved in public policy making and be politically active. Creating, influencing, and promoting legislation that improves a person's quality of life through home care should be a priority of all home care agency personnel. Also, home care should be on the forefront of providing a solution to the problem of indigent care. The efficiency of home care, coupled with its community health approach, may be a step toward resolving this issue.

CONCLUSION

Marketing provides the skills, the thinking, and the focus home health care agencies must have to survive and grow in today's competitive, changing, and challenging health care marketplace.

Home care administrators face numerous opportunities and challenges, such as generating adequate revenues and profits, providing clients with quality care, completing forms and reports accurately and in a timely fashion, and creating a positive environment of secure employment for themselves and their employees. It has been said that there is never enough time or money. This book is designed to help the administrator or marketer get more of both through the use of sound marketing principles. Marketing can help meet not only today's challenges and opportunities but also tomorrow's.

REFERENCES

Cetron, M. *The Future of Home Care.* Arlington, VA: Forecasting International, 1985 (released through the Foundation for Hospice and Homecare).

Cetron, M., O'Toole, T. *Encounters with the future: A Forecast of Life into the 21st Century.* New York: McGraw-Hill, 1982, 28-29.

Cole, R. The New Hospital. Speech presented at the Missouri Hospital Association Annual Meeting, Osage Beach, MO, November 6, 1986.

Griffith, E. The changing face of home health care. *Public Health Nursing.* 4(March 1987):1.

Griffith, E. Interview Elsie Griffith. *Family and Community Health.* 8(August 1985):77-80.

McCormack, M. *What They Didn't Teach You at Harvard Business School.* Toronto: Bantam Books, 1984.

Naisbitt, J. *Megatrends.* New York: Warner Books, 1982, 3-9.

Appendix

Market Plan

COMMITTMENT PHASE

1. Can management allocate the resources for developing a market plan?
2. Does management support the process of developing and implementing a market plan?

MARKET AUDIT

Market and Market Segments

1. Describe your market geographically.
2. How is your market grouped?
3. How do the following factors affect your market?
   Age of population
   Income of population
   Occupation
   Demographic shifts
   Geographic trends
   Seasons of the year
   Other
4. How many potential clients do you have?
5. How many of them are aware of your organization's services?

Organization

1. What is the basic philosophy of your organization?
2. What are the goals and objectives of your organization?
3. What are your organization's strengths and weaknesses? (See Worksheet A.)
4. Where has your organization's growth come from?
5. Where do you expect the growth to come from in the future?
6. How do conditions in other industries affect your organization?
7. What internal controls affect your organization?
   Advisory board
   Stockholders

WORKSHEET A
STRENGTHS AND WEAKNESSES

Item	Strengths	Weaknesses
Management		
Financial resources		
Staffing		
Facilities and equipment		
Services		
Image		
Reputation		
Other		

Board of directors

Staff

8. What external controls affect your organization?

Local

State

Federal

Self-regulation

9. What regulatory or legislative trends will affect your organization?

Client

1. What is the profile of present or potential users of your service?
2. How is your client profile different from that of the competition?
3. What is the frequency and quantity of client usage of your service?
4. Why do clients purchase or utilize your services?
5. Who makes the buying or utilization decision?

Competitors

1. How many competitors do you have?
2. Is this number decreasing or increasing?
3. Who are your principal competitors? (See Worksheet B.)
4. What is your competitors' share of the marketplace?
5. Is competition on a price or nonprice basis? (See Worksheet C.)
6. Where does the competition seem to be heading?

Services and Products

1. Analyze your services and products. (See Worksheet D.)
2. Are there any voids?
3. Do you plan to address these voids? How?

Pricing

1. What is the pricing philosophy of your organization?
2. How are the prices for services determined?

WORKSHEET B
COMPETITOR DATA

Organization name _____

Address _____

_____

Branch offices _____

Number of staff _____ Major clients _____

_____

Reputation and image _____

_____

Key personnel _____

Name _____

Title _____

Background _____

Strengths _____

_____

Weaknesses _____

_____

Pricing policies _____

_____

Marketing and promotional activities _____

_____

_____

_____

_____

_____

_____

WORKSHEET C
COMPETITOR ANALYSIS

List each feature or attribute of your agency and those of your competitors. Rate the the strength of each feature or attribute on a scale of 0 to 5 (0, lowest; 5, highest). Total each column to determine relative competitive strength or identify areas of potential vulnerability.

Feature or Attribute	Your Firm	Competitor 1	Competitor 2	Competitor 3	Competitor 4
24-hour nursing					
Occupational therapy					
Physical therapy					
Homemakers					
Trained staff					
Medicare					
Direct pay					
Total					

3. How do your prices compare with those of the competition?
4. How is your pricing viewed by

Client

Decision makers

Third-party payers

Organizations

Other

Promotion and Advertising

1. What is the objective of the organization's present promotional and advertising material?
2. How does promotional and advertising material support your marketing objectives?
3. What materials and activities will you use to create and maintain your image?
4. How are these materials and activities evaluated for results?
5. How are promotional materials and advertising integrated into personal selling?

Place

1. Where are you located in relation to your clients?
2. When did you last evaluate your present location?
3. What suppliers do you deal with?
4. What materials do you need on hand?

PLANNING PHASE

1. Is the problem identified? (See Worksheet E.)
2. Have goals been set?
3. Have objectives been developed?
4. Have strategies been developed?
5. Do the goals, objectives, and strategies address the opportunities identified in the marketing audit?
6. Is the final strategy selected?

WORKSHEET D
SERVICE AND PRODUCT ANALYSIS

Service or Product	Distinctive Features	Benefit to Client	How Viewed by Client	Total Cost	↑ or ↓	Why Heavily Utilized or Not

WORKSHEET E
PLANNING WORKSHEET

Problem: _____

_____

_____

Goal: _____

_____

Objectives: _____

_____

_____

_____

_____

_____

_____

Strategy ideas:

Strategy 1	Strategy 2	Strategy 3

Selected Strategy: _____

_____

IMPLEMENTATION PHASE

1. Do you have the acceptance of the target population?
2. What are the tasks necessary for implementation? (See Worksheet F.)
3. What resources and time frames are appropriate?
4. Is a control system in place?

CONTROL PHASE

1. Have the strategies accomplished the desired outcomes?
2. What modifications of the plan are necessary?

WORKSHEET F
IMPLEMENTATION WORKSHEET

Task	Resources	Due date	Done	Comments

Index

Administration commitment, 56
Adult day care, 217
Advertising, 10, 15, 16, 25, 60, 68, 72, 80,
    92, 130, 148
  word-of-mouth, 10, 25, 30, 35–36
Advisory board, 36
AIDA (attention, interest, desire, action),
    168
AIDS (Acquired Immune Deficiency
    Syndrome), 220
Alzheimer's disease, 154
American Association of Retired Persons
    (AARP), 36, 132, 154
American Hospital Association, 47
American Marketing Association, 205
American Medical Association, 16, 36
American Nurses' Association, 47
American Public Health Association, 47,
    203
American Red Cross, 23
Appearance, personal, 11, 169
Appointments, 162
Attitude, 10, 26, 27, 30, 73, 118, 156, 173
  multiattribute models, 28
Avon, 215

BARS (Behaviorally Anchored Rating
    Scales), 184
Baxter Travenol, Inc., 23
Beliefs, 27, 73, 94
  inferential, 28, 29
Beneficence, 204

Benefit(s), 16, 25, 33, 42, 44, 53, 81, 121,
    158, 171, 173
Blood drives, 35
Bonus, 174
Brochures, 140, 163
Budget, 50, 52
Business cards, 163
Buyer, 165

Cardinal Ritter Institute, 76
Case management, 43, 218
Categorical imperative, 203
Chamber of commerce, 46
Change, 13, 30, 88
  implementation, 103
  individual, 112
  resistance to, 102
  social, 214
Client, 10, 11, 15, 25, 32, 34, 44, 59, 68,
    77–81, 118, 119, 152, 154, 159, 216
  attitude, 73
  dissatisfied, 30, 34–35
  education, 73
  loyalty, 73
  profile, 77, 80
  sovereignty, 25–26
  surveys, 77–79
  usage pattern, 72
  values, 94
Clinical skills, 16
Close, 159
Closing, sales, 173

Cold calling, 163
Colloquialisms, 170
Commercial visitors, 150
Commission, 174, 183
Commitment phase, 56-62
Communication, 24, 56
  model, 129
  personnel, 109
  process, 129
  two-way, 148
Community activities, 35
Compensation, 183
Competition, 13-15, 45, 92, 160, 173, 180, 185
  analysis, 70, 80-81
Consultants, 42, 43, 174, 190, 193, 195-197
Consultative selling, 150, 151, 184
Consumer, 14
Content analysis, 210
Controls, 42, 44, 49, 53, 57, 77
  and evaluation, 44
Corporate culture, 206
Creating market plan, 49
Creative thinking, 197, 219
Customers, 7, 10, 12, 15. *See also* Client

Data collection methods, 116-119
  choosing, 116
  types, 116-118
Decision maker, 33, 148, 165
Demand, 93, 99, 211
Demographic, 65, 214
Differentiation, 8
Discharge planners, 15, 26, 30, 33, 36, 80, 81, 148, 150, 153, 155, 160, 161, 165, 171, 173
Disneyland, 12
Dissatisfaction, 34
Diversification, 90
Domino's Pizza, 12
Dress code, 31, 32
Durable medical equipment, 42, 84, 215

Economic conditions, 15
Economy, service-oriented, 11, 17-18
Elderly, 32, 47, 65, 76, 97, 132, 214, 217
Empathy, 153, 174
Employees, 13, 16, 22, 31, 43, 59
Entrepreneurs, 215
Environment, overall, 7, 211
Equipment, 157
Ethics, 13, 16, 34

Evaluation, 42, 47, 48, 123
  criteria, 118-119
  definition, 114
  effectiveness, 121
  efficiency, 119
  formative, 115
  program, 114-115
  purposes, 114
  summative, 115
Exchange, 4, 7, 23, 24
  complex, 25
  generalized, 24
  restricted, 24
Executive summary, 50

Facilities, 12, 76
Family, 27, 30, 34
Features, 11, 81, 171. *See also* Benefit(s)
Federal Trade Commission, 16
Feedback, 155, 157, 183, 198, 199
Fidelity, 204
Financial results, 17
First impression, 168
Focus groups, 31, 118
Follow up, 152, 159-161, 163, 172
Ford Motor Company, 14, 203
Foster Medical Corporation, 215
Foundation for Hospice and Home Care, 47
Future, 13, 16, 45, 51, 123, 194

Gantt chart, 52, 104, 106-107, 119, 120
Gatekeeper, 165
Goals, 7, 22, 42, 49, 50, 51, 57, 64, 115, 116, 123, 178, 182, 183, 199
  definition, 95
  examples, 95
Golden Rule, The, 203, 204
Gratitude, 204
Growth, business, 13, 14

Health Care Financing Administration, 90
Health fairs, 35, 141
Health planning model, 48
Homemaking services, 8, 25, 43, 132
Home parties, 144-145
Honesty, 205
Hospitals, 5, 6, 23, 32, 47, 148, 149, 155, 156, 161, 185, 191, 213, 215
Humana, Inc., 23

Identity, 13

Image, 6, 15, 17, 27, 32, 59, 76, 148, 150, 151, 155, 158, 159, 160, 163, 170, 183, 185, 206
  measurement, 30
Implementation, 44, 48, 102–112
  steps, 103
  strategy, 103
  worksheets, 104–108
    flow charts, 104–106
    Gantt charts, 105–106
    narrative, 106–107
Industrial Revolution, 4, 149
Influencer, 165
Initiator, 165
Innovation, 13, 215
Insurance companies, 216
Investment, 16, 17
Irresponsibility, 159

Joint Commission on Accreditation of Hospitals, 96
Justice, 204

Labor, 53
Labor unions, 216
Legislation, 212, 215
Lifestyle, 33
Listen, 109, 153, 169
Listening, *see* Listen
Location, 164. *See also* Place

Magazines, 35, 144
Mailing lists, 161
Management:
  by crisis, 180
  by objectives (MBO), 184
Market audit, 12, 36, 48, 50
  benefits, 64
  characteristics, 64
  definition, 64
  questions:
    advertising, 68, 72
    client, 68
    competitors, 68–70
    market, 66
    market segments, 66
    pricing, 68
    products, 68, 72
    promotion, 68, 72
Market development, 90
Marketer:
  characteristics, 194
  general skills, 194

qualifications, 193–194
Market information sources:
  formal, 45–47
  informal, 45, 47
Marketing:
  budget, 52, 60
  consultant, 195–197
  coordination, 44
  definition, 6–7
  era, 149, 150
  expenditures, 15
  history, 4
  goals, 48
  matrix, 98
  mix, 7, 11, 18, 148
  momentum, 198–199
  opportunities, 45
  orientation, 5, 6, 16, 56, 58
    self-study tool, 56–59
  planning, 58
    obstacles, 45
  purpose, 7
  responsibility, 43
    administrative considerations, 190
    in-house, 197–198
    organizational chart, 190–192
    outside consultant, 195–197
  strategy, 47, 48, 52, 90
    types of, 90
  team, 197–198
Market penetration, 90
Market plan, 22, 32, 44, 56, 179, 198, appendix
  phases, 49
Market planning:
  benefits, 42
  model, 48
Market segments, 132
  demographic, 65
  examples, 65, 72
  geographic, 32, 65, 84
  home health care, 72, 74, 75
  numerically, 65
Medicaid/Medicare, 9, 50, 72, 88, 90, 155, 156, 202, 212
Medical doctor, 26, 33, 148, 150, 153, 156–158, 173, 212. *See also* Physicians
Manager, 22
Membership lists, 161
Merchants, 149
Microeconomics, 8

Mission statement, 22, 131, 152, 161, 178, 182
Missouri Profile of Home Health Agencies, 77
Modification, 123
Morale, 15
Motivation, 174, 183
Muddling through, 179
Multiattribute attitude models, 28

National Association of Home Care (NAHC), 47, 94, 205, 212
National Center for Home Care Education and Research, 47
National health insurance, 212
National League for Nursing (NLN), 47, 93, 205
Needs, 4, 7, 16, 17, 27, 32, 53, 59, 181, 214
Nestlé, 203
Newsletters, 47, 142-144
News releases, 140
Nurses/Nursing, 25, 42, 43, 50, 59, 65, 73, 84, 109, 110, 149, 212, 213
Nursing home, 32, 154, 213, 214

Objections, 171
Objectives, 7, 22, 44, 49, 64, 115, 116, 123, 162
  definition, 95
  examples, 95-96
Open-ended questions, 155, 156, 171
Opinion leaders, 36
Opportunities, 51, 60
Organization, 73, 76-77
  components, 76
  philosophy of an, 73
Organizational buyer, 148
Outcome validity, 121

Pareto's law, 181
Partnership selling, 150, 151, 153, 184
Patient, 30, 48. *See also* Client
Peddlers, 149
Peer groups, 27, 34
Personality, 27, 33
Personal selling, 130-131
Personnel, 11, 17, 25, 30, 35, 110, 123
Physical:
  assets, 12
  facilities, 11
Physicians, 15, 23, 30, 34, 36, 48, 80, 81, 161, 171, 202. *See also* Medical doctor

Place (distribution), 8, 83-84, 92. *See also* Location
Planning, 42, 44, 88-89
  and change, 88
  models:
    exploitive, 89-90
    laissez-faire, 88-90
    types, 88, 89
  schedule, 44
  worksheet, 90, 91
Polaroid Corporation, 14
Portfolio analysis, 98
Positive reinforcement, 34
Power persuaders, 150, 173
Preparation, 163
Price, 8, 92, 155
  elasticity, 9
Pricing, 82-83, 205
Priority setting, 95
Problem identification, 91-95
Process management, 11-12
Procrastination, 179
Product, 8
  development, 90
Production era, 5
Professionalism, 151, 163
Professional meetings, 34
Promotion, 8, 9, 15, 92, 148
  and advertising, 83
  channels, 128, 129-130
  incentives, 131
  purpose, 128
  types, 83
Promotional messages:
  design, 132-133
  memorable, 136-137
  parts, 133-136
Promotional tools:
  advantages, 138-139
  characteristics, 137
  disadvantages, 138-139
  examples, 137-145
Prospecting, 181
Prospects, 161
Public health, 219
Public policy, 212, 219
Public relations, 6, 10, 60, 129, 148, 192
Purchase, 8, 33, 48

Quality, 10, 13, 23, 27, 31, 150
  of care, 5, 23, 32, 155, 180, 183
  of life, 23, 32, 213, 215, 217

Questions:
    closed-ended, 116–117
    open-ended, 116–117, 155, 156, 171

Random walk theory, 210
Recession, 213
Referrals, 34
Referral volume, 182
Regulation, 45, 215
Rejection, 183
Reputation, 14, 76, 151
Resource allocation, 42, 61
Resources, 42, 56
Retirement homes, 218

Salary, 174, 184
Sales, 7. *See also* Selling
    call, 161–173
    incentives, 10, 148
    people, 173
    resistance, 171
    training, 174
Satisfaction, 10, 15, 25, 34, 121
Self-improvement, 204
Selling, 5, 10, 59, 60. *See also* Sales
    era, 149
Seminars, 174
Sensitivity, 156
Services, 81–82
Sick day care, 33, 43, 94, 182, 215
Situational influences, 34
Social:
    change, 214
    costs, 82
    influences, 33
    responsibility, 202
Social Security, 212
Staff commitment, 57
Standards, 119
Strategy development, *see also*
    Marketing, strategy
    feasibility criteria, 96–97

types, 96–98
Stress, 169
Subordinates, 180
Success, 10, 11, 16, 17, 26, 47
Superwoman syndrome, 178
Surveys, 27, 30, 72, 122
Survival, 13–14

Target market, 7, 11, 32, 119, 185, 187
Teamwork, 59, 60
Telephone, 46, 159
    etiquette, 31
Television, 35
Territory:
    analysis, 182
    managment, 180–183
Third-party payers, 8, 24, 32
Time, 17, 158
    management, 178
    nonproductive, 181
Travel, 53, 181
Trend impact analysis, 45
Trends, 210
Trust, 183
Tuberculosis, 218

United Way, The, 57
User, 165
Utilitarianism, 203

Value, 24
Values, 7, 27, 33
Video tapes, 141–142
Visiting Nurses Association (VNA), 131,
    134
Visiting Nurse Service of New York,
    210

Wants, 7
Word-of-mouth advertising, 10, 25, 30,
    35–36
Workshops, 142